PRAISE FOR *PATHWAYS TO PREGNANCY*

"What a wonderful contribution Mary Wong has made to women
and couples facing the challenges of trying to get pregnant.
Warm, approachable, and professional, she skillfully guides
readers through the benefits of using the best of both Western
and traditional Chinese medicine in dealing with conception
challenges. Her book is filled with honest but encouraging accounts
of how these two practices can work in concert with each other
to help women achieve their dream of becoming mothers."

TONI WESCHLER, AUTHOR OF BEST-SELLER
TAKING CHARGE OF YOUR FERTILITY

"An inspirational account of personal stories
of women triumphing over infertility."

REBECCA FETT, AUTHOR OF *IT STARTS WITH THE EGG*

"In *Pathways to Pregnancy* Mary Wong tells her own and other
couples' stories of fertility treatment, whilst offering advice
based on the best of both Eastern and Western medicine.
Anyone struggling to conceive will find this a helpful book."

JILL BLAKEWAY, LICENSED ACUPUNCTURIST, CO-AUTHOR OF
MAKING BABIES, HOST OF CBS RADIO'S *GROW. COOK. HEAL.*

"Written by a thoughtful, compassionate practitioner,
Mary Wong's *Pathways to Pregnancy* offers solace and hope to
everyone called to travel the 'scenic route' to parenthood."

JULIA INDICHOVA, AUTHOR OF *INCONCEIVABLE* AND *THE FERTILE FEMALE*

"Moving, inspiring and full of hope for women navigating the often heartbreaking journey of infertility, Mary shares the stories of her patients and her own personal infertility experience with an authenticity that will give comfort to all those trying to conceive."

RAY RUBIO, DOCTOR OF ACUPUNCTURE AND ORIENTAL MEDICINE, EXECUTIVE DIRECTOR OF THE AMERICAN BOARD OF ORIENTAL REPRODUCTIVE MEDICINE

"As an acupuncturist and former embryologist, I know too well that fertility goes beyond fertilizing an egg and a sperm. If you or your loved ones are struggling with fertility and want to know how to optimize your chances, this book is an invaluable resource. Mary Wong provides a superb A-Z fertility guide, combining years of professional experience with her personal journey to take you to a deep level of healing and transformation that can very well be the missing piece in achieving your pregnancy."

HELEN BETGIVARGIS, FORMER IVF EMBRYOLOGIST, FOUNDER OF ACUPUNCTURE TREE OF LIFE

"Mary Wong is the only person I know who could create such an effective amalgam of Eastern and Western approaches to fertility care."

DR. MARJORIE DIXON, MD, FERTILITY SPECIALIST, FOUNDER AND CEO OF ANOVA FERTILITY & REPRODUCTIVE HEALTH, ASSISTANT PROFESSOR AT THE UNIVERSITY OF TORONTO

"Pragmatic and expressive, Mary Wong shares real stories about human infertility, and weaves into them her vast knowledge of Eastern medicine as well as Western medicine, which together amount to a real 'human medicine.' Reading these tales, you can't help but be reminded of similar journeys that you or those you know have taken. In all of this, a clear Mary Wongian philosophical truth emerges: that there is definitely more water in the glass than you can possibly imagine!"

PAUL TUREK, MD, UROLOGIST AND MALE REPRODUCTIVE HEALTH SPECIALIST, FOUNDER OF THE TUREK CLINIC

"This landmark book gives readers not only a sense of direction, but a sense of belonging and community. Often, couples and individuals trying to make sense of their struggle feel incredibly isolated and misunderstood. And this feeling is not without merit, because so few of us have loved ones who can truly relate to the emotional torture that fertility issues can bring. Mary Wong shares heartfelt stories that embody the journey beautifully, and that will bring true hope and healing to many."

CHRIS AXELRAD, LICENSED ACUPUNCTURIST, PAST PRESIDENT OF THE AMERICAN BOARD OF ORIENTAL REPRODUCTIVE MEDICINE

"Mary's book offers a nurturing way of healing for those struggling with infertility. This is a must-read for anyone wanting to take back control over their fertility journey. I will be recommending this book to my patients."

"Combining the best of Chinese medicine and Western medicine, Mary draws on her personal wisdom and extensive patient experience to forge a path to overcoming infertility that will inspire and support you on your journey to pregnancy."

Pathways to Pregnancy

Personal Stories and Practical Advice
for Your Fertility Journey

Mary Wong

R.TCMP, R.AC

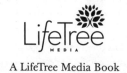

A LifeTree Media Book

Published by
LifeTree Media Ltd.
www.lifetreemedia.com
Distributed by
Greystone Books Ltd.
www.greystonebooks.com

Cataloguing data available from Library and Archives Canada
ISBN 978-1-928055-16-7 (paperback)
ISBN 978-1-928055-17-4 (epub)
ISBN 978-1-928055-18-1 (pdf)

Editing by Lynne Melcombe
Cover design by David Drummond
Interior design by Ingrid Paulson
Printed and bound in Canada
Distributed in the U.S. by Publishers Group West

The information contained in this book is not intended to serve as a replacement for professional medical advice. Any use of the information in this book is at the reader's discretion. The author and publisher specifically disclaim any and all liability from the use or application of any information contained in this book. A health care professional should be consulted regarding your specific condition. The stories in this book are true. Subjects' names have been changed to protect their privacy.

To all women and men who walk this path:
May you discover hope, healing, and miracles.

Table of Contents

Foreword

As I read this book, one primary message came through to me: hope. Hope for women facing fertility challenges is woven into every word. What a great relief women experience when they can share stories of their difficulties, their journey, and what they learned during the process. In my experience, women heal most deeply when they can tap into and accept their own vulnerability by hearing what others have gone through.

When I began experiencing fertility challenges, I knew something was wrong but was only familiar with Western medicine. I didn't know anyone else who had gone through the lonely and often frustrating hopelessness I was feeling. I had never been exposed to Chinese medicine, and when first introduced to the possibilities of traditional Chinese medicine (TCM), I found them strange—I simply could not fit this approach into my logical brain. Yet, it worked. The changes in my body and mind, the awakening of my heart and spirit were irrefutable, yet inexplicable. I had to study this healing modality and find out what made it work.

In the years since then, I have devoted my life to the practice of TCM—learning, practising, teaching, and offering it to many thousands who suffer through their own devastating fertility challenges. I met Mary Wong in the early years of my teaching, and she made a strong impression. It's always a bit intimidating for a Westerner to stand in front of a Chinese doctor, attempting to share my view of a medicine that was part of her cultural upbringing.

Mary was undoubtedly knowledgeable, but what struck me most about her were her honesty and openness. She is the kind of person who not only makes a good doctor but a trusted friend. She rode the interface between Eastern and Western culture and medicine, devouring knowledge, learning and treating, studying, serving, and giving it all she had. In her clinic, people healed. And when she went through her own fertility struggles, like me, she was down and dirty with the psycho-emotional component. "Physician, heal thyself" were not mere words to Mary; she lived them.

Mary can do what I have never quite pulled off, and her abilities are evident in this treasured book you hold in your hands. There is a beautiful image in Chinese philosophy of an organic life form rising from the very substance of earth itself, embodying the spirit of creation in its impulse to walk, breathe, and experience the miracle of this life as it reaches toward the light of its own existence. It is richly Asian, conveying through imagery what TCM offers. Mary's effortless expression of who she is and what she was born to do is apparent in the ease with which she conveys the power of Chinese healing, while at the same time demystifying it with her concise understanding of modern Western science.

When I was interning in a Chinese hospital, I was tired and overworked, and my energy and immunity were low. Yet like a typical American overachiever, only semi-conscious of the messages my body was giving me, I pressed on. One day, an attending physician took my pulse, and the next day I was served soup for lunch with the Chinese herbs I needed to restore my energy. While I thought it odd that food and medicine be combined in one dish, this is Mary's starting point. It's in her bones.

Fertility struggles are frustrating and isolating. They seem to eat away part of a woman's soul. They can plunge a woman down to the depths of her despair, but they can also force her to face difficulties in the way she's living her life. I can think of almost nothing else that can do this. Yet sometimes, when we're in our lowest places, where we feel nothing can pull us out of the muck, true healing can happen. This is a place of courage and honesty that few are lucky enough to know. And where a woman's body had been saying "no" to life, it can ever so gently turn into a "yes." This is what I call hope. If you want to find this hope, it's important to know you are not alone. There is support. There is another way.

I wrote *The Infertility Cure* many years ago, attempting to open up this new way for women who were locked into the often frustrating approach of reproductive medicine. Mary picks up where I left off, walking you along a pathway she herself has trod. With wisdom, honesty, and a lighthearted pragmatic approach, she blends modern Western science with the ancient art of Chinese medicine. Hand in hand with you, she shares poignant real-life stories of help, hope, and true healing. Her unending positivity as she counsels and comforts you along the way is infectious: may you catch it and make it part of your journey.

Randine Lewis, PhD, L.Ac
Author of *The Infertility Cure*
and *The Way of the Fertile Soul*

Introduction

Since I was a young girl, I've known I wanted to make a difference in people's personal lives and have been strongly drawn to
fields involving health and well-being. Initially, I planned to go
to medical school. I did not come from a long line of traditional Chinese medicine (TCM) practitioners. In fact, when I
was growing up, I shied away from anything to do with my
Chinese heritage.

Having been born in the Netherlands, lived in Hong Kong,
and then moved to Canada by the time I was eight years old,
I wanted nothing more than to blend in with the neighbour-
hood kids. Embarrassed when my parents spoke Chinese to
me in public, I spoke back to them in English. My mom would
call me a bamboo star (Asian on the outside but culturally
hollow inside) or a banana (yellow on the outside and white
inside). Maybe it was fate that led me back to my roots as I
witnessed first-hand the miracles of acupuncture and Chinese
medicine.

It was the summer of 1988. I had just finished my second
year at McMaster University, where I was studying biology.
My eighty-six-year-old grandmother became very sick and we
took her to the local hospital. At first, the doctors thought she

had cancer, but her biopsies came back negative. I remember sitting behind the drawn hospital curtains, using nail clippers to cut off the hardened skin peeling away from the palms of her hands like scales. It was difficult to watch her wasting away in front of me.

Just as I finished and she lay sleeping, the doctor in charge came in and told us her kidneys were failing, but he did not want to operate due to her age. He gave her two weeks to live. Grief came over me; I was very close to her. She lived with us and had always taken care of us growing up, as my parents had worked long hours in the restaurant business. But I held it together for her sake. There was nothing left to do but bring her home and make her as comfortable as possible in her dying days.

Then my older brother said, "We're Chinese. Perhaps we should try Chinese medicine?" He looked up a TCM doctor in the Yellow Pages (a print directory everyone used before computers and websites came along). I drove her to Chinatown for treatment by a renowned TCM doctor, who must have been in his seventies himself. After three weeks of acupuncture and Chinese medicinal soups, she started to feel better. Within three months, she regained her health and her energy. I marvelled at her miraculous recovery and became disenchanted at how easily she'd slipped through the cracks of mainstream medicine, which had pronounced her as good as dead.

After I finished my university degree, instead of applying to medical school, I went on to learn the art and science of traditional Chinese medicine (TCM). Since then, I've made it my life's mission to bring about change and improve people's health by bridging the gap between Eastern and Western medicine. In my first ten years of practice, I realized my dream by joining forces with Dr. Jess Goodman, a family physician who invited me to open up the first integrative medical practice in Mississauga, a city in the Greater Toronto Area. For over two decades, I've had the privilege of guiding countless patients back to wellness by combining Eastern and Western medicine.

Throughout that time, I've had a fire burning inside me to write this book, to share my story and other stories of miracles I've observed through my clinical practice and personal experiences—stories of men and women whose remarkable recoveries after negative mainstream diagnoses have defied what's understood about modern science.

At the core of our existence is the undeniable and natural desire to create life. Every year, however, millions of people around the globe face fertility challenges. TCM practitioners generally see everything, and in the course of my practice some of those people found their way to my clinic. By word of mouth, people learned that I treated fertility successfully and compassionately. Moreover, I did not get married until I was thirty-eight, and having a child was always in the back of my mind, so it interested me to preserve my own fertility. Over time, as my TCM practice grew, so did the portion of it devoted to fertility challenges. At this point, I've seen it all: the heartbreak, the grief and shame, the hope, and the joy of eventual pregnancy and childbirth.

Traditional Chinese medicine is the oldest experiential science in the world. This ancient wisdom has been tested through the ages, and documented directly from patient response. For thousands of years, TCM doctors discovered what worked and what didn't, and continued to expand upon knowledge accumulated through acupuncture and Chinese herbal medicine.

These are not the kind of double-blind studies on which modern Western medicine bases its treatment of sick patients. However, Chinese medicine is the world's largest and longest study of how to prevent and treat illness, conducted on real people for thousands of years. All the drugs in the world combined have not been tested to this degree.

Stemming from the philosophy of Taoism, which means "the way," TCM emphasizes living in harmony with nature and being in the present. It's a holistic practice incorporating acupuncture, Chinese herbal medicine, lifestyle, exercise, and proven dietary therapies. The strength of Chinese medicine comes from its focus on preventing illness. In the days of the Emperor, his physician was paid only when the Emperor was well and not if he was ill. Only royalty and the very wealthy enjoyed the privilege of access to the Chinese doctors' expertise.

Today, in Western culture, we are not taught to maximize our health and prevent illness as we're growing up. Most of us were raised with the Western medical model, which focuses on examining individual parts of the body and treating illness affecting these parts. If we have pain, we typically take anti-inflammatories and painkillers. We tend to wait until something goes awry before we treat it. We do not learn other things we can do and other health practitioners we can consult who specialize in preventive health care. We learn to take better care of our cars than ourselves; for example, we know we need to change the oil and take our vehicles for regular tune-ups. But when it comes to health, many people put their bodies in the hands of their doctors instead of seeking the knowledge and insight to know and feel when their system is out of balance.

I don't mean to generalize, as many patients I see are proactive in their efforts to conceive—curious and interested in doing whatever they can to prepare their bodies, minds, and spirits for having a healthy baby. However, most of my patients come to me as a last resort, often desperately seeking help because they've already been having difficulties getting pregnant, often for months or years. Many of my patients have said they wished they'd come to my clinic first, before embarking on the expensive and painful journey through fertility clinics.

This book includes stories, both instructional and inspirational, for anyone experiencing infertility or seeking to understand it. These stories offer hope, humour, and a healthy dose of practical advice—advice that is often overlooked by mainstream practitioners but easy to incorporate into your life. The stories are real, although I've changed the names, and sometimes the occupations, of the women and couples I've written about to protect their privacy. My hope is that these accounts of their fertility struggles will inspire you to take charge of your reproductive health and overall well-being.

One of the best things you can do for yourself when trying to get pregnant is to focus on yourself—to relax and be in the moment rather than focusing your energy on trying to put a baby in your belly. Through your fertility journey, you will find there is no one "right way" to build a family, but there is a way that's right for you.

The inward focus demanded by the drive to procreate necessitates a holistic and intuitive combination of Western and Eastern medical traditions, plus a huge dose of love and self-acceptance. A strong foundation of balance and aligned energy enhances the possibility of conception. By blending new research in the field of *epigenetics* (which I will discuss more in Chapter 1) with experiences from Eastern and Western medicine, *Pathways to Pregnancy* can help you optimize your chances of conceiving while nourishing the unborn mother in you. Rather than dealing alone with the overwhelming amount of contradictory information online, *Pathways to Pregnancy* can help you navigate the fertility world, dispel your shame, decrease your stress, discover the surprising interconnectedness of life, and renew your belief that you can overcome fertility challenges.

That said, I do not want to create false hope. In practice, I always say, "I cannot guarantee a baby in your belly" and "We cannot force a pregnancy; we can only encourage it." Whether you are trying to conceive naturally, with the help of assisted reproduction through a fertility clinic, or with a combination of both, it's up to nature to decide if there will be a pregnancy.

My insights into this increasingly common condition go beyond the professional. I myself went through a long process of fertility treatments, eventually conceiving and giving birth to my daughter Zoe in 2012. I write at some length about this in Chapter 8. The point is, I am more than a practitioner handing out advice to those struggling with infertility; I have "been there" myself, I know how patients feel, and this knowledge has made me a better and more empathetic TCM practitioner.

You may be tempted, when reading this book, to skip over chapters you think don't apply to you. For example, if your fertility challenge is rooted in poor ovarian reserve, you may wonder why you should bother with the chapter on PCOS. However, I encourage you to read every chapter, for several reasons.

First, each chapter includes at least one and sometimes two inspirational stories. For women and men with fertility challenges, the pathway to pregnancy can be stressful; you need all the inspiration you can get. Second, many of the sidebars in the book are pertinent to the whole topic of fertility challenges, not just the particular issues addressed in the chapter in which they appear.

Similarly, although each chapter focuses on a particular problem, it also includes information that anyone facing fertility challenges could find helpful. For example, although Chapter 5 focuses on male factor infertility, it includes information about a gender bias in the fertility world that virtually every woman experiences. And through the remarkable story in Chapter 9, I pose the question, "How far would you go?" It's a question all women, men, and couples should consider early in their fertility journey, and this chapter illustrates why.

Whether you are just thinking about starting a family or have been struggling with fertility challenges for years, *Pathways to Pregnancy* offers real hope of healing. More than that, it may be useful for your friends, family, co-workers, and employers as they strive to support you in your journey. Finally, it may help those who hope to start a family someday by informing them of what can go wrong and encouraging them to use TCM to be proactive in caring for their own reproductive health.

And it all started with my grandmother. If she had not fallen ill, I might never have taken an interest in Chinese medicine, and I might not be telling you my story now.

By the way, she lived another eight years and died at the age of ninety-four.

1

You Are Not Your Diagnosis

A woman is like a tea bag; you never know
how strong it is until it's in hot water.
ELEANOR ROOSEVELT

Vanessa: Unexplained infertility

Vanessa met her husband, Robert, at thirty-two, married at thirty-four, and started trying to have a baby right away. After six months, they went to her family physician to get a referral to a reproductive endocrinologist (RE). Couples must have tried to conceive for at least a year without success to be referred to a fertility specialist. For some, every passing month feels like an eternity. This must have been the case for Vanessa, who fibbed to her family doctor, telling her they'd actually been trying for a year.

At the same time as Vanessa was seeing the RE, she was coming to my clinic for acupuncture. I encourage my patients to get medical testing if they're having trouble conceiving because it provides a baseline from which I can help them more naturally align themselves and their environment to support conception. It also allows us to rule out any structural or genetic issues.

Through my TCM examination, I discovered Vanessa had premenstrual symptoms, including several days each month of breast tenderness, back pain, lower abdominal pain, weakness, and moodiness. Like many patients who have visited a fertility clinic, Vanessa was surprised by the depth of my inquiry into all aspects of her health and lifestyle. At the fertility clinic, her diagnosis of *unexplained infertility* was based solely on her report of not becoming pregnant despite trying for a year and the clinic's inability to find an explanation. Her RE advised her to begin treatments as soon as possible because she was thirty-five—approaching what fertility clinicians call *advanced maternal age.*

A jumping-off point

One of the most difficult things I see in my clinic is a woman who is in her mid-thirties, still feeling young and vibrant, yet distressed after a fertility doctor has used terms like "unexplained infertility" and "advanced maternal age."

I greatly respect fertility specialists; as I discuss in Chapter 8, my own daughter was born through IVF. I've experienced the stress of fertility clinics first-hand, as well as the miracle of birth using *assisted reproductive technology* (ART). The difficult part is healing the emotional impact of a diagnosis on my patient's body, mind, and spirit.

I have my work cut out for me when a healthy thirty-five-year-old is weeping in my office, having been told to consider *intrauterine insemination* (IUI) and *in vitro fertilization* (IVF) before her aging eggs reach their expiration date. My first job in this situation is to shrug off my own anger at a doctor who would say such cold words to a woman who's come seeking help.

I am not suggesting you ignore your diagnosis, or live in denial of it, but that you think of it as a jumping-off point, an opportunity to become proactive in your fertility journey and overall health. You are a dynamic human being; with a renewed perspective, you and your body can both change. Do not let a doctor's words stop you. Your pathway to pregnancy may just be different than the one you had planned.

White-coat hypertension

There is a well-known effect called *white-coat hypertension or white-coat syndrome*. This is when a patient whose blood pressure is normal when monitored at home becomes elevated at the doctor's office. Just sitting in front of a doctor can cause emotional anxiety and raise your blood pressure. I well remember my heart racing and my palms sweating on my first visit to a fertility clinic.

I tell patients that a blood test captures conditions at a moment in time. During those initial visits, a woman is at her most vulnerable— nervous, anxious, and worried. If her doctor says he doesn't expect she can get pregnant naturally and she'd better start treatments right away, she may feel sadness, despair, grief, anger, frustration, fear, worry, and anxiety. Worse, she may barely have time to take in this information and process her emotions before feeling pressured to choose her next steps.

I felt all of these emotions over the course of my own fertility treatment, and I want to share with you how important it is to acknowledge, process, and release them. Words from a physician are powerful and can elicit strongly negative emotional, psychological, and physiological impacts. This is called the *nocebo effect*, Latin for "I shall harm," a term coined by Walter Kennedy in 1961.[1]

I see the nocebo effect every day in my clinic. Many patients believe a doctor's words are the absolute truth, but that diagnosis represents a particular doctor's beliefs and theories, based on experience, statistics, and research. Without intending to discount these, any doctor's knowledge of research can be outdated, and their experience is necessarily confined to their own practice.

Over the years, I have seen many women who have undertaken extensive fertility treatments go off on their own, whether to take a break from treatments or stop entirely, and spontaneously conceive. It happens too often to be written off as coincidence.

You have a filter

The first step in hearing your diagnosis in a healthier way is to change the filter through which you hear it. This is not simple, and it's not likely to happen overnight, but you can start by becoming aware that you have a filter and paying attention to its impact on your ability to remain positive. Here are some ways you can change your filter:

- Ask yourself, is your diagnosis the ultimate truth? When I received my diagnosis (see Chapter 8), I acknowledged the condition but refused to live with the label "infertile." Instead, I opened myself to creative ways of building a family, including IVF, donor eggs, and adoption. At the same time, I continued with my healthy diet, moderate exercise, and positive lifestyle.
- Surround yourself with positive people.
- Be grateful for your overall health.
- If the doctor says you are reproductively old, find examples of women who defy the odds and tell yourself you can be one of them. (I hope you will find yourself in some of the women I describe in this book.)
- Remind yourself that the tests form a baseline picture of your current reproductive health. Focus on what you can do to improve that picture by taking charge of your diet, lifestyle, and stress-management strategies.
- Remember that a diagnosis is usually more opinion than fact; you can always get a second opinion.

Pregnancy really is a miracle

We see pregnancy around us so often that we take it for granted. Few of us realize how many conditions must line up perfectly just to prepare a woman's body to conceive. Consider this simplified list of requirements for an embryo to become implanted:

1. The brain (hypothalamus, pituitary) must release the right hormones properly to stimulate egg development.
2. An egg of good enough quality must develop to maturity, and it must be chromosomally normal.
3. The brain must release *luteinizing hormone* (LH) to stimulate final ripening of the egg and *ovulation* (release of the egg).
4. The follicle in which the egg develops inside the ovary must rupture at time of ovulation and release the egg.
5. The fallopian tube must "pick up" the egg.
6. The sperm must be of good enough quality to survive and swim up the fallopian tube from the vagina and through the cervical mucous.
7. Once there, the sperm must sit ready and perched, waiting for the egg to drop so it can penetrate the shell.
8. The sperm must release its DNA of twenty-three chromosomes into the egg to fertilize it.
9. The fertilized egg must undergo cellular division to become an embryo and then continue to divide normally.
10. The embryo must make its way down the fallopian tube into the uterus by the third day of development, where it will have a different environment in which to survive and grow.
11. Once there, the embryo must continue to develop and expand into a *blastocyst* (a multi-celled embryo) and then hatch out of its shell and implant in the uterus.
12. The endometrial lining of the uterus must be ready for implantation (a complicated, multi-step process of its own).

Western medicine and fertility clinics focus on what might be wrong with any of these details, how they might explain it, and how they might fix it. They test blood levels of reproductive hormones and examine ultrasounds of developing follicles. They administer hormones; perform IUI, IVF, or surgeries; or combine these technologies.

TCM looks less at the details and more at the big picture. After all, women's bodies have been going through this intricate process for millions of years. According to TCM, when the conditions are right and your internal environment is balanced and healthy, your chances of conceiving and carrying a healthy and successful pregnancy to term are great.

What is "unexplained infertility"?

Infertility is defined, in Western medicine, as when a woman has been unable to conceive after a year of unprotected sex. When a doctor can't find a specific explanation for this, he or she may diagnose *unexplained infertility*. Twelve percent of couples experiencing fertility challenges are diagnosed with unexplained infertility.[2]

I see women nearly every day who have spent months conscientiously trying to conceive, feeling hopeful and excited. They've also had monthly feelings of disappointment and sadness when they discovered they weren't pregnant, whereupon most resolutely return to baby-making. But many of the women in my practice admit to going online and diagnosing themselves with unexplained infertility after only a few months of unprotected sex.

Please don't do this. It has a negative impact on your ability to keep a positive state of mind. I rarely use the word "infertile" in my clinic. In my opinion, this word alone can create a negative environment in your body, mind, and spirit. It's a word I've spent many hours counselling my patients to stop focusing on.

Unfortunately, when a woman hears a diagnosis of infertility, she infers, "I am infertile." My perspective is that, at that moment in time, that woman's system is simply saying, "No, not now" to having a baby. Instead of using the words "infertility" or "infertile," I encourage women to say, "At this time, I am having a challenge with my fertility."

In my practice, I have seen many women conceive outside of the one-year time frame. The only fertility challenge I diagnosed was that they were out of balance and needed guidance to create a nurturing environment and prepare their soil to receive and nurture their seeds.

How TCM can help

One of the first things I do with patients who've been diagnosed as infertile is to help them let go of their negative assumptions. Acupuncture sessions may help them release thoughts and feelings that seem stuck in their minds, while counselling or hypnosis may help them process upsetting experiences they've had on their journey to conceive.

What you can do with any TCM practitioner is optimize your chances of creating life by treating underlying imbalances that Western diagnostic tools may not reveal. TCM goes beyond technological diagnoses to look at your overall state of health by inquiring into your lifestyle habits and your physical, emotional, and psychological well-being. The philosophy in Chinese medicine is that you are most likely to conceive naturally when you are more balanced physically, mentally, and emotionally.

Using Chinese medicine, I guide my patients to achieve balance in their overall well-being rather than focusing on the twelve tiny details of implanting an embryo or the specific challenges their body is going through. Throughout this book, I will share with you the same guidance I share with them about eating healthier, engaging in moderate exercise, relaxing, and creating a positive environment in which to grow a baby.

Blending Eastern and Western medicine

Vanessa and I began weekly acupuncture treatments—at the same time as she went to her fertility clinic—to help dissipate and rectify her imbalances. Although her menstrual cycles were regular at twenty-eight days, her other symptoms, according to TCM, reflected imbalances within her cycle.

Western medicine focuses on the numbers associated with menses. It considers a menstrual cycle irregular if it is less than twenty-five or more than thirty-five days; twenty-eight days is considered normal. In TCM, however, we also consider the quality of menses and associated symptoms, like the number of days of blood flow; the thickness, colour, and odour of the blood; and the extent of abdominal pain and bloating, fatigue, and headaches before, during, and after menses.

In TCM, these details reflect a woman's overall state of health and degree of balance within the environment in which she hopes to grow a baby. The information I gather provides a baseline for the way a woman's body and reproductive system are functioning. I provide information to help my patient better align her body to receive life. For Vanessa, I did acupuncture at specific sites with the goal of sending a message to her brain to release certain hormones, while inhibiting others to decrease her menstrual symptoms and improve her reproductive balance.

Vanessa chose to monitor her cycle through the fertility clinic. Beginning on the third day of her cycle, the woman returns to the clinic almost daily for blood tests and a *transvaginal* or *intrauterine ultrasound,* in which a technician inserts a *transducer* (phallic-shaped probe) covered with a condom and lube into the vagina and blood tests. The ultrasound counts the number of *antral follicles* (ovarian follicles that contain eggs) the woman has and tracks their growth, while the blood tests measure hormone levels.

Initially, these tests may be performed every couple of days, increasing to daily as the time for ovulation approaches. The woman may also receive injectable hormones to incite *super-ovulation,* which stimulates the ovaries to create more than one egg, increasing the chance of conception. Cycle monitoring and injectable hormones prepare the woman for timed intercourse or IUI. During IUI, a catheter deposits *pre-washed sperm* (the normal and denser sperm, which is separated by a centrifuge from the semen and less viable sperm) directly into the uterus. (Think of it as the turkey-baster method.)

Vanessa immediately underwent three consecutive rounds of cycle monitoring with injectable hormones, followed by IUI. She conceived after the first IUI, but the pregnancy only lasted a few days. This is termed a *chemical pregnancy* as there was nothing visible to show she was pregnant. After two more IUI cycles without conceiving, Vanessa was disappointed, but the one positive pregnancy test gave her the courage to have a small uterine *polyp* (benign growth) removed in case it was a factor in preventing implantation.

After the surgery, Vanessa and Robert decided to try IVF. Although she conceived the first time, it was an *ectopic pregnancy,* which occurs when the fetus develops outside of the uterus, typically in one of the fallopian tubes. She then had to wait several months before trying IVF again. After the second IVF, she conceived again, but the fetus had *trisomy 18*, a chromosomal abnormality, and Vanessa miscarried in the second trimester. She waited another six months before trying a third IVF, which was unsuccessful.

Using TCM to balance your life

At this point, nearly four years had passed since Vanessa and Robert first visited the fertility clinic. She'd had several IUI cycles and three IVF treatments, and had taken countless fertility drugs. During this time, Vanessa would come to my clinic for treatment but then disappear for long stretches of time. Often women take breaks from treatment, sometimes to mourn the loss of a baby through miscarriage.

After one of her breaks, Vanessa came to me for a relaxing acupuncture treatment and caught me up on her journey. She felt frustrated, like nothing she did was ever enough, she couldn't make the right choices, and things were out of her control. She worked hard to control the things she could, such as what she ate and drank.

We talked about how even eating and drinking must happen in balance. Many women I see obsess about their food intake, convinced that eating a spotlessly healthy diet will boost their chances of conception. Vanessa wasn't giving herself much leeway; at her mother's birthday she felt bad for not eating any birthday cake. When her mother said one piece wouldn't kill her, she took a small piece but felt guilty about cheating. Imagine the stress of thinking a single piece of cake could ruin her chances of conceiving, thus wasting all the time, money, and effort they'd already invested. This is just not the way it works!

In Chinese medicine, we believe in living a balanced life. We expect you to eat and drink in order to nourish yourself physically, emotionally, and spiritually. If you have cut gluten, sugar, and dairy out of your diet and feel deprived, I say you are out of balance. Perhaps, instead of depriving yourself, you could consider healthier treats. For example, instead of a Mars Bar, you could buy some organic dark Belgian chocolate and eat with reckless abandon once in a while.

Eating for fertility: What to eat

The following tips will not only create a better environment for conception but will help you grow a healthy baby too:

- In general, pick easy recipes with simple ingredients and choose whole, unprocessed, high-fibre foods.
- Make soups with bone broth, ideally homemade. Bone

marrow contains precursor cells for red and white blood cells. In TCM, the marrow is considered Jing essence, or kidney energy, which controls reproductive energy. Some people consider beef bones superior because the marrow is more concentrated, but they must also be cooked longer. With more and more people avoiding red meat, I recommend chicken bones and cartilage. Regardless, all bone marrow is very digestible yet filled with minerals (calcium, magnesium, potassium, and phosphorus), as well as good fats and simple proteins. (See sidebar on page 14 for a recipe for chicken bone broth soup.)

- Eat organic foods where possible to avoid pesticides and additives, which have been shown to cause menstrual irregularity, miscarriage, stillbirths, and developmental defects, as well as reducing fertility and increasing time-to-pregnancy.[3]

- For lunch and dinner, fill half your plate with cooked vegetables, such as spinach, zucchini, leeks, string beans, lettuce, sugar snap peas, Swiss chard, carrots, alfalfa sprouts, peppers, artichokes, cucumbers, asparagus, dill, avocado, eggplant, bamboo shoots, escarole, sauerkraut, beans, seaweed, beets, onions, cilantro, parsley, garlic, mushrooms, okra, tomatoes, olives, celery, water chestnuts, peas, and ginger root. These vegetables help keep the body alkaline, creating a healthy environment for sperm to thrive.[4] They also provide lots of nutrients, including vitamins A, C, B6, B12, K, beta carotene, calcium, vitamin E, folate, iron, niacin, copper, magnesium, manganese, phosphorus, potassium, zinc, omega-3 fatty acids, and selenium, all of which are vital to your overall health as well as to making a baby. Veggies are also good sources of dietary fibre, which keeps your bowels healthy and regular.

- In addition to the above vegetables, eat plenty of cruciferous vegetables, such as bok choy, kale, broccoli, Brussels sprouts, cauliflower, cabbage, collard greens, turnips, and radishes. Research has shown cruciferous vegetables help to detoxify carcinogenic cells and reduce oxidative stress. In TCM, these vegetables are believed to help the liver cleanse your body of toxins (which is its primary role in our bodies) and excess hormones (which may accumulate during fertility treatments).

- Eat iodine-rich foods. Eating only cruciferous vegetables can reduce your iodine levels, which are essential to proper thyroid function, and thyroid function is essential to hormone production. You can counteract this by eating dried sea vegetables such as seaweed, wakame, hijiki, dulse, kombu, and kelp. In addition, Himalayan Crystal salts, cod fish, plain yoghurt, boiled eggs, navy beans, cranberries, strawberries, and supplemental iodine can keep your iodine levels healthy.

NOTE: Do not supplement with iodine or eat too much iodine if you have a diagnosis of *Hashimoto's disease,* where your body attacks your own thyroid gland, which is responsible for releasing hormones into your body. If in doubt, minimize iodine-containing foods, as an excess can be bad for your health, but consult a health care practitioner with extensive knowledge of supplements.

- Diversify your food intake to maximize nutritional benefits from a variety of different foods.
- Drink one litre of hot water with the freshly squeezed juice of one whole lemon as your first drink of the day. This gently wakes up your stomach, which decreases inflammation,[5] aids digestion and eases constipation,[6] eliminates toxins (by virtue of moving your bowels), calms anxiety by acting as a natural antidepressant,[7] and helps with weight loss.[8] Lemons also contain ascorbic acid, which protects sperm

DNA and prevents oxidative stress.[9] Think of juicy water-filled cells!

- Buy non-genetically modified foods (non-GMO) so you know they are derived from nature and not saturated with man-made pesticides.
- Eat protein at every meal because proteins are the building blocks of life. Protein sources include:
  > Lean organic meats, like skinless chicken.
  > Vegetable-based proteins in the form of legumes and nuts, such as chickpeas, lentils, split peas, quinoa, beans, nuts and nut butters (especially walnuts and almonds), sunflower seeds, hemp seeds, sesame seeds, poppy seeds, almond milk, and hemp milk. Eggs are a good source of protein, but make sure they're from free range, organically fed, antibiotic- and hormone-free chickens.
  > Fish. Smaller species are better as they are likely to have absorbed less mercury, lead, and other heavy metals, which can disrupt immune function and subvert the body's ability to receive an embryo.[10] They can also affect the reproductive system and can be toxic to the growing fetus via the placenta,[11] posing a health threat to the developing brain and possibly leading to low birth weight and size.[12]
- Eat plenty of foods containing omega-3 fatty acids. Essential fatty acids (EFA) are naturally anti-inflammatory, and the older we get the more inflammation we tend to have in our bodies (kind of like rusting). The best EFA (DHA and EPA) are found in fish, but it's important to stick with those with the lowest contaminant levels, such as wild salmon, Arctic char, Atlantic mackerel, sardines, sablefish (black cod), oysters, anchovies, rainbow trout, and mussels. Olive oil, garlic, flax seed, walnuts, dark leafy greens, cabbage, and Brussels sprouts contain another EFA called ALA. The body converts

ALA to DHA and EPA, which are vital in pre- and post-natal brain and behavioural development.[13] As well, one study showed fertile men had higher levels of EFA as compared to infertile men;[14] this is known as a correlation rather than a causal relationship, but there are plenty of reasons for all of us to increase our EFA consumption. As well, for women, EFA appear to help with embryo quality.[15]

Chinese herbal chicken bone broth

Start with 1 large whole chicken, about 3 pounds (organic, free-range, hormone- and antibiotic-free). Preheat oven to 350 degrees Fahrenheit. Drizzle chicken with olive oil and rub all over with sea salt and pepper. Into the cavity, insert 1 lemon cut in half, 2 sprigs of thyme, a bay leaf, and some sprigs of rosemary or sage. Roast for about 1 hour. After 30 minutes, baste with cooking fluids and then baste every 10 minutes until done.

In the meantime, fill your largest stock pot with cold filtered water and add the following organic vegetables:

2 large carrots, peeled and cut in half
3 celery stalks
1 tomato cut in half
1 large onion cut in half
2 tbsp of apple cider vinegar

Add the following Chinese herbs, which you can pick up at any Chinese herbal dispensary or Chinese grocery store. Wash them before adding to the stock pot:

- Gou Qi Zi or Goji berries (lycii berry or wolfberry fruit)—a large handful. (Choose the less bright red ones to be sure no colorants have been added.) In TCM, Gou Qi Zi is believed to nourish the blood and kidneys, lower blood sugar, have antioxidant properties, prevent fat build-up in liver cells, and help regenerate liver cells.

- Shan Yao (dioscorea or Chinese wild yam)—3 pieces. In TCM, Shan Yao is believed to nourish digestion, nourish kidney and reproductive energy in men and women, regulate menstruation, lower blood sugar, soothe mood, aid sleep, and benefit overall blood and qi energy.
- Huang Qi (astragalus root)—3 pieces about the size of a tongue depressor. In TCM, Huang Qi is considered an overall tonic that regulates blood sugar and enhances sleep, energy, and libido, as well as the immune system and metabolism.
- Bai Shao Yao (white peony)—2 pieces. In TCM, Bai Shao Yao is thought to nourish the blood, soothe the liver, soothe abdominal cramps, and nourish nutritive (yin) energy. It is used to help with endometriosis, ovarian cysts, and menstrual cramps, and to regulate menstruation.
- Hong Zao (dried Chinese red jujube dates)—3 pieces. In TCM, Hong Zao is believed to calm the nervous system, inhibit cell mutation, protect the liver, improve energy, and have an antihistamine action, which benefits the immune system.
- Fu Ling Poria—3 pieces. In TCM, Fu Ling Poria is believed to aid and strengthen digestion, decrease water retention, reduce stomach acid, calm the heart, soothe the nerves, and sometimes help with insomnia.

When the chicken is cooked, slice off most of the meat for dinner, but cut the leftover meat into bite-sized pieces and store in the fridge. Put all the bones and skin into the stock pot and bring to a boil. Lower to a high simmer so there is minimal bubbling, and cook for 12 hours.

If you need to leave the house, you may need to take it off the stove and store it in the fridge while you're gone. Alternatively, you may leave it simmering in an electric crock pot for 12 hours.

With a slotted spoon, take out all of the chicken pieces, herbs, and vegetables, and place them in a sieve over a large bowl to collect any stock that drains from them. Discard the pieces from the sieve and strain the rest of the stock through the sieve.

Drink a cup per day. Or cool and pour into separate containers to freeze and use for cooking or as a soup base.

To make chicken soup, heat the stock and boil with 2 peeled and diced carrots, 2 cut celery stalks, and 1 diced onion. Add some parsley and season with salt and pepper to taste. Before serving, add in cut up chicken bits from the roasted chicken.

Eating for fertility: What not to eat

Keeping your body fit to receive an embryo and grow a healthy baby is not only about what you put into your body but also about what you keep out of it. The most important foods to avoid include:

- Sugar, especially refined white sugar, but also fruit juices. Sugar of all kinds can cause blood glucose to spike. This can increase insulin resistance and cause ovulatory issues and impede fertility.[16] Research has shown that sugar is more addictive than cocaine in its effect on the reward centre in the brain—the more you eat, the more you want.[17]
- Artificial sweeteners, as they increase inflammation and can negatively affect the growth of eggs, especially for women with *polycystic ovarian syndrome* (PCOS; see Chapter 6).
- Prepackaged, factory-canned, and boxed foods with long expiration dates, which includes things like commercial chocolate bars, boxed mac-and-cheese, and canned pasta with tomato sauce. Packaged foods are convenient but are also filled with chemical flavourings, colourings, artificial ingredients, preservatives, and fillers. Even the packaging

itself is sometimes questionable (for example, plastic contains carcinogens, and there is some concern they may be released when heated).

From a TCM perspective, the above guidelines are common sense for anyone wishing to maintain a healthy inner environment. The following suggestions are more specific to improving fertility.[18]

- Fast foods and fried foods that contain excessive trans-fatty acids (TFA), which can potentially increase insulin resistance.[19] This, in turn, can increase weight and impede ovulatory function, decreasing fertility potential. TFA are widely known to be unhealthy fats.
- Gluten-containing foods, which may disrupt hormone function, increase inflammation, tend to be higher on the glycemic index (which lists foods according to their impact on blood sugar), and increases body fat, which can disrupt ovulation.[20] A diet with too many foods high on the GI can also increase insulin resistance, which I will discuss more in Chapter 6. If you are sensitive to gluten, a diet high in gluten can cause inflammation and activate autoimmune disorders (see Chapter 7), which can contribute to miscarriage.[21]
- Meats containing growth hormones and antibiotics, which can disrupt your natural hormonal balance.
- Fruits grown with pesticides. Eat organic as much as possible, since toxins can disrupt hormonal balance, but particularly avoid fruits such as peaches, pears, apples, grapes, celery, spinach, and strawberries if they're not organic. Refer to the most updated list created by the Environmental Working Group (EWG), which ranks pesticide levels on produce tested by the U.S. Department of Agriculture and the U.S. Food and Drug Administration.[22]

- Alcohol. If possible, abstain altogether. I often see women who drink moderately, and if they have a negative pregnancy test, they have a drink; that is unlikely to affect their chances of conceiving in the future. However, a Danish study showed that women over thirty who consumed more than one drink per day were more likely to have fertility issues than women who consumed less than one drink per week.[23]
- Coffee and caffeine-containing teas and sodas. It's best to reduce caffeine intake to less than 200 mg per day. Research has shown that two cups of regular coffee or five twelve-ounce cans of caffeinated soda can double risk of miscarriage.[24] However, it's difficult to assess how to keep within that 200-mg limit when another study found that twenty different commercial espresso coffees exceeded the maximum safety limit in just one cup (they contained from 200 to 322 mg per shot).[25]
- Dairy products, which contain insulin-like growth factor (IGF-1), especially when taken from high-producing milk cattle.[26] IGF-1 at high levels can increase insulin resistance, which can in turn affect proper timing of egg maturation, especially for women with PCOS (see Chapter 6).
- GMO soy products. Even for non-GMO soy products, do not exceed sixty grams (that's three twelve-ounce glasses of soy milk) per day. Soy contains *phytoestrogens* (plant-based estrogens), which can upset hormonal balance.

Eating for fertility: How and when to eat

There is more to healthy eating than what you physically stick into your mouth. It is just as important to nourish your mental, emotional, and spiritual well-being as to eat a healthy diet. In TCM, this includes how and when you eat (and don't eat). My aim is to put joy back into your eating experience while boosting your fertility. (NOTE: If you have celiac disease, are lactose intolerant, or have any known food allergies or intolerances, you will want to stay away from whatever you react to.) The following simple guidelines will help you look and feel better inside and out:

- Eat lightly cooked vegetables, as they are readily digestible (partially digested by the cooking process) but not over-cooked to the point of losing nutritional value. Steaming or stir-frying vegetables lightly helps your digestion and enables your body to extract nutrients more effectively.
- Chew your food thoroughly. Breaking food down before it goes into the stomach helps the process of digestion.
- Try an eating meditation where you take a bite of your food, chew it well, slowly, and consciously (preferably with your eyes closed), noticing the textures and flavours in your mouth.
- Do not multitask while eating, as you might normally do. Just eat and breathe and notice the calmness that arises as you practice being present during your meal. You may even notice that this style of eating helps your digestion, since normally you may not chew your food as thoroughly and may gobble things down too quickly.
- If you are following a specific dietary regimen, treat yourself once in a while (ten to twenty percent of the time) without worrying about it. If chocolate is your vice, buy organic chocolate and enjoy every morsel. If you love the ritual and taste of coffee, drink a small cup of organic coffee once or twice a week. Make treating yourself a meditative and soul-ful experience. Ironically, as you begin to eat healthier foods, your taste buds may become more sensitive and, when you give in to a craving, the food may not taste as good as you imagined. That piece of chocolate cake with ice cream may taste sickly sweet and make you feel bloated. The good

news is you can make your own treats and control the quality and quantity of the ingredients (like sugars).

- Stop judging what you (or others) are eating. Eating something "bad" does not make you a bad person. This type of self-judgement is tied directly to guilt and shame, both of which can negatively impact your physical, mental, and emotional well-being, and affect the environment into which you hope to grow a baby.
- Share and enjoy food with others. Humans in most cultures have been eating communally since the beginning of time. Sharing food with family, friends, and colleagues affects your natural healing response. It brings more relatedness, laughter, and joy to your life, which leads to physiological, psychological, social, spiritual, and quality-of-life benefits.[27]
- Eat at regular intervals and do not skip meals; this will help keep your blood sugar levels balanced.
- Prepare and eat home-cooked meals as much as you can. This allows you to control the ingredients in your food. It also enables you to make extra food to freeze in meal-sized containers for when you don't have time to cook properly. You can also cook fresh vegetables, but make enough for two days. If you find it's difficult to cook during the week, make several recipes on the weekend that you can eat and freeze. If you need to resort to take-away food sometimes, choose health-conscious establishments, avoid deep-fried foods, and make special requests such as adding more vegetables and decreasing high-carb foods.

NOTE: Often, my patients complain to me about the cost of organic food, yet not too long ago it was considered normal for the average family to spend forty percent of their income on food.[28] In 1901, the U.S. Bureau of Labor Statistics, Consumer Expenditure Survey found that families from New York and Massachusetts spent 42.5 percent of income on food.[29] Now it seems we want to spend less on food and more on material goods like cell phones and computers. Perhaps it's not that organic food is too expensive, but that you might consider re-evaluating the cost of your health.

Vanessa's spontaneous miracle

Having undergone several IUI and IVF cycles, Vanessa and her husband were taking a break from the stress of fertility treatments, although Vanessa was still doing acupuncture at my clinic and eating a balanced diet. She and her husband felt they had exhausted the technological resources in their hometown of Toronto and were researching the Colorado Clinic of Reproductive Medicine (CCRM) in Denver. They thought the CCRM offered more advanced testing than the Toronto clinic she was attending, and Vanessa and Robert met with the fertility doctor to discuss this option.

After the meeting, Vanessa noticed she had some spotting, although her period wasn't due for five days. She joked with her husband that her ovaries were reacting to the sound of the fertility doctor's voice and got scared into getting pregnant in order to avoid another IVF. What she didn't know was that the spotting was implantation bleeding. A few days later, she couldn't ignore the symptoms anymore; she'd been pregnant so many times that she was completely in tune with her body.

"It was three o'clock in the morning and it sort of hit me," she told me later. "I got up and did a pregnancy test in the middle of the night. After four years of trying to conceive, I was pregnant with Mia." What surprised her most was that her husband had been away for work that month and they'd only had intercourse once, well before ovulation.

A woman's fertile window is about five days before ovulation, and on ovulation day. After ovulation, the window of receptivity to sperm is twelve to twenty-four hours. The idea is to try to have sex before ovulation, allowing the sperm to swim up to and sit in the fallopian tubes, where they can live up to a maximum of seven days ready and waiting for the ovulating egg. This must have been what happened when Vanessa finally became pregnant—the old-fashioned way, with no technology.

2

The Everywoman of Fertility Challenges

It does not do to dwell on dreams and forget to live.

J.K. ROWLING, *HARRY POTTER AND THE SORCERER'S STONE*

Avery: Poor ovarian reserve

Avery was a hard-working, goal-oriented woman. At thirty-six, having achieved partnership in her law firm, she focused on her goal of having two children before she reached forty. After two years of trying to conceive with her husband of seven years, they sought help from a fertility clinic. After undergoing IUI unsuccessfully, she attended my clinic feeling desperate and frustrated.

Avery's first impression of my TCM clinic was that it was calm, restful, welcoming, and warm, in contrast to the necessarily sterile medical environment of the fertility clinic. She sat on my treatment table, commenting on the comfort of the pillows and sheets in contrast to the disposable paper at the medical clinic. When our conversation turned to her unsuccessful IUI, however, her tears began to flow.

I encounter this almost daily in my practice. The women who come to me feel more than devastated; they feel broken, as if their inability to have a child negates every area of their lives—lives in which they are not only competent but sometimes very accomplished. I provide a safe space for much-needed emotional release. I told Avery there was nothing I could say to ease her pain. There's no other way to describe it except to say it's unfair, and, well, it sucks.

I call this the mourning period, a time to grieve the loss of a wanted child. In Chinese medicine, we view this as a healthy and necessary emotional purge. It's important and healthy to experience your emotions and get them out rather than trying to bottle them up inside and get on with your busy life.

The seven affects of emotions

In Chinese medicine, we recognize the need to experience the "seven affects" of emotions. It is a healthy and necessary part of the human experience to express joy, sorrow, worry, grief, fear, fright, and anger. When we harbour and suppress these feelings over a prolonged period without expressing or purging them, we give rise to disharmony, which affects our physical well-being, including our fertility.

Infertility myths

Before coming to my clinic, or going to a fertility clinic, Avery and her husband had tried to conceive on their own for twelve months. After six months of having sex three times a week without conceiving, Avery used an *ovulation predictor kit* (OPK) from the local pharmacy to time their intercourse during her peak ovulation times. She would pee on a urine stick every day from eight days after her menstrual period began; when a happy face appeared on the pee strip, it indicated her most fertile time (when her surging luteinizing hormone triggered the release of a mature egg from one of her ovaries). This peak indicated the small window of opportunity each month in which she might conceive, typically about six days.

Avery, an overachiever, said she and her husband would have intercourse daily, sometimes twice, to "get the job done." She admitted their love-making had become mechanical, timed, and devoid of spontaneity. Instead of focusing on their connection and mutual enjoyment, she strategized the best sexual position to maximize conception; after he gave his "sperm donation," she'd stick a pillow under her bum and lie on her back with her feet propped up against the wall. She'd stay in that position until morning, not even peeing before she slept so no semen would leak out.

Like most of my patients, Avery avidly read books and online information about enhancing chances of conception. Collecting information from so many, sometimes conflicting sources, leads many women to gather unhelpful advice that can even interfere with conception.

Holding your urine may seem like a good idea, but you run the risk of a urinary tract infection (UTI), especially if you are prone to them, as Avery was. Also, by "holding it in," there is a natural tendency for the pelvic floor to tighten and constrict, which can be counterproductive to conception.

Moreover, it's a myth that the sperm readily "leaks out." Sperm are dynamic; it's unavoidable that some get left behind, but the dynamic sperm quickly separate from the seminal fluid as they swim up to the fallopian tubes. Once there, they may sit for several days waiting to fertilize a matured egg as it descends from one of the ovaries.

The fertility clinic experience

After twelve months of trying on their own without success, Avery's family doctor referred her to an RE at a fertility clinic in Toronto. Avery described the process as impersonal and stressful. At their first consultation, she and her husband gave blood samples and spoke briefly with the doctor before being ushered to separate rooms for preliminary tests.

Avery was shown to one room for a trans-vaginal ultrasound. The technician watched a monitor attached to the probe while moving it inside Avery's vagina, looking inside her left and right ovaries for the developing antral follicles as well as examining the thickness of the uterine lining. This invasive process, which every fertility patient undergoes, can be very uncomfortable, but is necessary to determine the state of your fertility in that moment and therefore the likelihood of IVF success.

At the same time, Avery's husband, Walter, was led to a small room just big enough for an armchair, a TV with a DVD player, and a small collection of X-rated movies and magazines. He was handed a plastic specimen cup and told to produce a sample. Fifteen minutes later, he handed his sperm sample to the nurse to be tested.

Avery and Walter then met briefly with the doctor, who described their next steps, and talked about statistics and probabilities. Typically, the fertility doctor shares Western medicine's facts and perspectives about fertility, often without having seen their test results. For a woman who is already feeling emotional, vulnerable, and stressed, the process can feel dehumanizing.

In a nutshell, the doctor told Avery and her husband that, reproductively speaking, at thirty-eight, she was old. They should start right away with cycle monitoring, where the clinic would track her ovulation and they would be directed to have intercourse at the optimal times. Their chances would be moderately better if they came to the clinic for IUI. If that didn't work for them after three tries, they could try IVF. But they should decide quickly because Avery's eggs were "getting older by the day." So she returned to the fertility clinic on the third day of her menstrual cycle and for many mornings thereafter for early morning *cycle monitoring* (CM).

Leading a busy life as a partner in a law firm and not wanting to be late for work, Avery would go to the fertility clinic before dawn each morning in an effort to put her name down first on the sign-up sheets at the reception counter. One list was to check the hormone levels in her blood, the second was to look at her developing follicles through trans-vaginal ultrasound, and the third was to meet with the doctor.

Somehow she never managed to be first. By 7 a.m. daily, the waiting room would be full of women seated quietly with their heads in a book or their cell phones, avoiding contact with each other. Avery preferred the anonymity, and dreaded the thought of running into someone she might know. A private person, she worried about admitting to someone she was having trouble conceiving.

Mentally prepare to go to a fertility clinic

If you are reading this book before your first visit to a fertility clinic, the information in the next section will help you prepare for it. If you have already been to a fertility clinic, and it was as difficult for you as it is for most women, this information might help you put your experiences into a different perspective.

Even if you don't plan to go that route, you have no way of knowing whether your own pathway to pregnancy will end up taking you there. As a mother who didn't plan to use a fertility clinic but ended up doing so, I can promise that you don't always know where your fertility journey will take you. Although this section will equip you with information I give patients who come to me before attending a fertility appointment, it's information you may find useful no matter where you are on your pathway.

An opportunity to gather information

I counsel my patients to view the fertility clinic as a step on their path, and I suggest you see it as an opportunity to gather medical information about your current baseline reproductive health. Along the way, remember you are always in charge. When it comes time to make decisions, pay attention to your intuition. Attending an appointment at a fertility clinic does not bind you to undergoing any kind of interventions.

Create a positive state of mind before attending your first appointment. Fertility doctors typically compare your test results against what they believe to be the "norm." But you are a dynamic individual, capable of change, and your body has an innate way of healing itself. Use the tips and techniques you'll learn in this book to take an active role in your reproductive health.

Please do not consider the fertility doctor's diagnosis to be the final word. Their evaluation is an educated guess, an opinion based on statistical averages and numbers. Each woman is unique. Many babies are born despite unfavourable diagnoses from fertility specialists.

The clinic doctors may speak in generalizations. If you are over thirty-five, your fertility doctor may say you are reproductively old. If your tests indicate your eggs look less than stellar, remember that this test represents a moment in time. Eggs are cells that develop over the course of a year. From a TCM perspective, you can have a profound impact on your eggs' health in their last ninety to 120 days, while they are growing and proliferating, by making positive changes in your life. Fertility doctors are not versed in TCM principles and do not view egg health as flexible, but as we'll see in Chapter 5, egg health can change dramatically in a short period of time.

If you have already been to a fertility clinic

If you have already been to a fertility clinic and found it diffi-cult, try to reframe your visit with these thoughts in mind: It was an opportunity to collect baseline information about your reproductive health. Your doctor's opinion is just that—an opinion. You are not bound to follow any advice that makes you uncomfortable and you need to listen to your intuition in making decisions. Your visit may have left you feeling out of control, but you can take back control any time you choose. Your first step may be to try TCM as a way of getting a second opinion from a different perspective.

Epigenetics and environment

Before learning TCM, I studied sciences and was always looking for ways to demystify this ancient Chinese art. Even after I entered practice and was helping countless patients achieve their goals of better health and healthy babies, I continued to seek modern explanations for the centuries-old success of Chi-nese medicine.

Reading about quantum physics, which recognizes the energy fields or "Qi" that we study in Chinese medicine, excited me, but when I heard Dr. Bruce Lipton, a renowned cellular biologist, speak at an acupuncturists' conference in 2004, his words and research resonated with me in a profound way. Dr. Lipton discussed the new science of *epigenetics*, a complex cellular science that says environment affects the health and well-being of our cells even more profoundly than genetics. Even our conscious and subconscious thoughts, beliefs, and emotions are part of our environment.

For me, Dr. Lipton's work was the missing link, helping me understand why in TCM we focus on harmony and balance of body, mind, and spirit as the foundation of all health. Moreover, what we think, feel, and believe about our environment affects our health and, in this case, fertility.

Dr. Lipton says a "cell's life is controlled by the physical and energetic environment and not by its genes."[1] In my TCM world, everything I do with my patients is intended to help them heal and balance their physical environment, using acupuncture, herbs, and diet to alter their energetic environment, encourage positive thinking, and pay attention to thoughts, feelings, and beliefs.

At the very foundation of fertility are two cells: the egg and the sperm. The largest cell in a woman's body is her egg and smallest in a man's body is his sperm. Everything I discuss in this book relates to how I help my patients create a nourishing, healthy, balanced environment in their bodies, minds, spirits, and surroundings to give their cells, especially their eggs and sperm, the best possible chance of developing into life.

Nature's balance

Traditional Chinese medicine helps us understand how to restore and preserve balance in the body, mind, emotions, and spirit. Once balance is restored, and environment is optimized, many women in my practice achieve spontaneous conception. TCM stems from observing nature and viewing our bodies as microcosms of nature. We believe we must cultivate the earth before we plant the seed.

In nature, life erupts from fertile ground in supportive environments. In my clinic, we use TCM principles to create the ideal physical and energetic environment to increase the chance of conceiving a baby. In my experience, when the conditions are right in body, mind, emotion, and spirit, life happens spontaneously. When we go off course, our internal homeostasis becomes unbalanced. Some women's bodies tell them of imbalance through frequent bouts with the flu, sore muscles, colds, or headaches. Other women's bodies alert them of imbalance by presenting fertility challenges.

The work of the TCM practitioner, then, is to determine the causes of the imbalance and offer workable solutions to correct them and restore the body to a naturally healthy and balanced state that's right for conception. TCM recognizes that our internal and external environments affect this balance. What we eat and drink; how we think, feel, and live our lives; and what we are exposed to in our environment all affect our overall well-being.

Western fertility clinics focus attention on gathering a patient's medical history, blood tests, ultrasound results, and sperm analysis. Fertility doctors factor in a woman's age to calculate her odds of having a healthy baby, and say they can improve those odds by using modern treatments and technologies. While some women have been told to reduce their stress and lose weight to increase their odds of conceiving, I have never heard of a patient whose RE told her to pay attention to the physical and energetic wellness of her internal environment because it would affect her eggs and her partner's sperm.

For the first month after their initial visit to the fertility clinic, after having her cycle monitored, Avery and Walter had timed intercourse. It was more accurate than self-testing by peeing on a stick because the technician visually tracks the growth of the egg and follicle, and checks hormone levels via bloodwork. The nurse called, directing them to have sex as Avery would be ovulating within the next day or so.

Avery's test results

Timed intercourse is the most basic intervention a fertility clinic offers. They administer no drugs, just monitor eggs and hormone levels so intercourse can coincide with ovulation. Unfortunately, Avery did not become pregnant this way. So a month after their first visit, Avery and Walter returned to meet with the doctor. The good news was that Walter's sperm count was good: he had 100 million sperm per millilitre, well within the normal range of 20 to 300 million. Avery, however, was devastated to learn that, as a woman over age thirty-five, she had poor ovarian reserve (POR) and they would likely need greater intervention to achieve pregnancy.

Although the doctor said they could try a round of IUI, he warned them not to waste time and recommended they move straight to IVF before Avery "ran out of eggs." Or perhaps, he suggested, they should use donor eggs from a younger woman, fertilized with Walter's sperm. He offered these options while handing them a brochure for their donor egg program, which Avery interpreted as, "You are over the hill in terms of trying to get pregnant."

Avery was in shock. She'd gone to the fertility clinic seeking hope and encouragement, and instead felt old, broken, and depressed. How could her eggs be too old when she had regular periods, was healthy, active, and looked younger than her age?

They decided to try an IUI cycle with a hormone medication called Letrozole to increase their odds of getting pregnant by releasing multiple eggs at ovulation. She produced two eggs, which the doctor said would double her chances of conceiving.

For two weeks after the insemination, Avery convinced herself she was going to have the baby of her dreams. After she went into the fertility clinic for an early-morning blood test, she waited anxiously by the phone for the results of the pregnancy test. Every passing minute felt like an eternity.

When she received the phone call that afternoon, the nurse apologized and told her the blood test had come back negative: she was not pregnant. She would need to return to the fertility clinic on the third day of her menstrual cycle to start cycle monitoring again. Instead, Avery came to my clinic.

What is poor ovarian reserve?

There are three main markers of poor ovarian reserve (POR):

- High *follicle stimulating hormone* (FSH). FSH is a hormone released by the pituitary gland (which is in the brain) to stimulate the growth and maturation of follicles and the eggs within them. Measuring a woman's blood levels of FSH on day two or three of her menstrual cycle tests her ovarian function. If her FSH levels are above ten, it suggests she is approaching menopause because her ovaries are working harder to produce eggs. High FSH means the woman would respond poorly to IVF because FSH is the drug used to stimulate egg production.[2]

- If FSH is already high, adding more FSH will not help. Think of cooking with gas. You release gas to turn on the flame and start cooking. To a point, you can turn the gas higher to speed up the cooking. But after a certain point, more gas and a higher flame won't help the cooking process; it will just burn the food. Similarly, in a woman's body, adding more FSH will help stimulate egg production to a point, but after that point, it will actually make things worse.

- High FSH was once considered a key marker of POR, but we now know that FSH can go up and down over time, which makes it less reliable as a marker of infertility. That said, it is a reliable way to determine how women are likely to respond to FSH drugs. If FSH is normal, they're likely to respond well; but a high FSH indicates a poor response to stimulation drugs for IVF since these drugs use FSH.

- Low anti-mullerian hormone (AMH). Until recently, women were thought to be born with their lifetime supply of ova (immature eggs), which secrete AMH. (Research has now shown egg precursor, or stem, cells in the walls of the ovaries of mice[3] and women,[4] dispelling this belief.) The amount of AMH in a woman's blood, which remains constant throughout her menstrual cycle, is considered a good indicator of the quality and quantity of remaining eggs in her ovaries, and therefore a better measure of ovarian reserve than FSH.

- That said, AMH levels are considered controversial, because it's unclear how accurate or cost-effective it can be at predicting live births or improving reproductive health care, and there's a lack of international standards for interpreting test results accurately.[5] And personally, I have witnessed some women's AMH improve with treatment.

- Low *antral follicle count* (AFC). AFC is the number of follicles visible on day three of a trans-vaginal ultrasound. Each antral follicle contains one immature egg, which potentially develops and is released by the ovaries during ovulation. AFC indicates a woman's ovarian reserve, expected response to ovarian stimulating drugs, and chance for successful pregnancy through IVF.

- For IVF, the more antral follicles visible to stimulate with hormones from the third day of menstruation, the greater the chances of having them all mature so they can be retrieved surgically through the vagina and become fertilized in a petri dish. More follicles mean potentially more embryos and a greater likelihood of conception.

What TCM thinks of your "old" eggs

When Avery started trying to have a family at thirty-six, like many women her age, she believed she had lots of time to have a child. She began worrying about her age when, at thirty-eight, she still hadn't conceived. Unfortunately, her fertility doctor did not provide comfort or reassurance. When she came to see me, she was not only upset that she hadn't conceived after her first IUI but was still troubled by the things her doctor said at their first appointment. She didn't know how to get past the statistics the doctor had presented and she admitted to having negative thoughts and feelings that were interfering with her ability to stay positive.

Instead of talking about biological age as markers for fertility, in TCM we speak about fertility in terms of our vitality and energy. In the ancient practice of TCM, we believe we are born with a certain amount of energy, which we inherit from our parents. This finite amount of energy is referred to as Jing Qi (primordial, congenital, source energy, or Essence). In addition, we are able to tap into and produce energy through food and drink, which TCM refers to as Gu Qi (acquired nutritive energy). We also acquire energy from the air (oxygen) we breathe and metabolize it into usable energy for our bodies. This includes energy for procreation. While we can replenish the nutritive Gu Qi, our Jing Qi declines with age and living.

Women's energetic life stages

Chinese medicine goes on to say that women and men have energetic stages in their lives. For women, these stages are in cycles of seven years (for men it's eight):

- At seven, a girl's Jing essence (her inherited energy) becomes bountiful and manifests in permanent teeth and healthy hair.
- At fourteen, she enters puberty as her essence fills her reproductive organs and menstruation begins.
- At twenty-eight, her sexual energy peaks.
- At thirty-five, her sexual essence begins to decline. Jing Qi energy is divided into different functions, which includes sexual energy/essence.
- At forty-nine, a woman's reproductive essence becomes exhausted and menopause ensues.

According to Chinese medicine, a woman's procreative energy is not accessible indefinitely, but neither does it end at thirty-five or forty years of age. We acknowledge the shift in her reproductive essence at age thirty-five but believe that a woman who lives in balance with nature in body, mind, and spirit can spontaneously conceive right up until the onset of menopause. My two grand-mothers both had healthy babies at the age of forty-six.

TCM believes that, as we age, we deplete our Jing essence. The more we over-extend ourselves, the more we deplete this essence. Stress is a major cause of this depletion: working long hours for years on end is physically draining; hating your job and feeling unfulfilled is emotionally and spiritually draining.

Also in TCM theory, the fertility journey, if not approached in a balanced way, can deplete your energetic essence. Anyone who has faced fertility challenges will attest to how taxing they can be phys-ically, emotionally, and spiritually. The key is to mitigate your stress and conserve your energy, including the sexual energy required to create life.

Achieving balance through TCM

After Avery and I talked about the different perspectives TCM and Western medicine have of reproductive health, we addressed the importance of creating balance in her world. That included processing and letting go of the things her fertility doctor told her to expect, or not expect. When a woman who is working hard at conceiving hears that, statistically, her efforts may be in vain, that kind of information can stick—especially when her fears are being confirmed by a doctor in a lab coat.

While Avery understood the TCM concept of energy and essence, she was still convinced she was going to have a chal-lenge conceiving because her fertility doctor told her so. But because the environment in my clinic is so different from the fertility clinic, and my staff and I were welcoming, nurturing, and attentive, Avery began to open up to the possibility that the fertility doctor did not have the final word. I assured her that I would not make false promises, but that given her history and health, I believed she could become pregnant. Avery decided to work with me and my team for three to four months with a view to creating an environment in which she and her husband could make a baby.

Avery expressed to me in our initial meeting that she was worried she'd waited too long and on some level regretted pursuing financial stability, career, and partnership in her law firm. She wished they'd tried when they were younger instead of avoiding pregnancy so diligently. She was beating herself up for past choices. I encouraged her to let go of these negative thoughts, reminding her that they did not contribute to a healthy environment into which to welcome a baby.

Socio-economic trends

Having access to birth control for the past several decades has prevented women from having unplanned pregnancies, allowing young people to focus on education, career, and financial stability and delay marriage and childbirth. One study showed a thirty percent increase in women in the skilled work force from 1970 to 1990.[6] Along with this, women are working more hours. There is also a self-incentive to delay marriage and childbirth because of the known "family gap" in the workplace, where a working mom generally receives less pay than a childless woman.[7]

In 1972, women comprised thirty-eight percent of the general workforce,[8] and today it has increased to nearly half in the United States[9] and Canada.[10] Fifty-one percent of employed women work in management and professional positions,[11] which tells me that as many women as men are in the workforce and as many working women as working men are in stressful, demanding jobs with long hours.

I will talk more about work stress in Chapter 6. The important point here is that there is no blame. In a world of rising living standards, modern women invest in and focus on their education and financial security. Focusing on the next promotion or achieving seniority can make it difficult to even contemplate finding a mate or making babies. Even in relationships, both partners generally work and, with busy schedules, often struggle to find time for intimacy. As a result, a woman's natural maternal instincts can be set aside and suppressed as she is consumed by demands of work.

Survival mode kicks in

Avery and I discussed the years of stress she'd been under, first working toward partnership and then trying to conceive. That kind of stress can create disharmony and imbalance in the body. And being a high achiever, Avery's workload and stress continued now that she had a financial stake in the firm.

She and her husband had started trying to have a baby immediately after she'd achieved partnership. They'd not prepared at all for a baby, other than not using protection. And each month when her period came, she shoved aside the emotional stress of not being pregnant, which in and of itself can be an emotional rollercoaster ride of hope and anticipation, followed by sadness and despair. This alone can be so overwhelming as to perpetuate long-term disharmony in the body.

According to TCM, when your body goes through cycle monitoring and even a single IUI cycle, as Avery's did, your system becomes taxed. If you've already accumulated a lot of stress in your life, these procedures can send your system into survival mode, where your ovaries and uterus are almost dormant as your energy is diverted to support your brain, heart, and limbs. This does not mean your body is failing you, but that it is lovingly and protectively telling you, "Not yet. Let's wait for a better time, when you are in a more balanced state physically, mentally, and emotionally, before becoming pregnant."

After I explained to Avery the impact on her fertility of the years of stress she'd endured, she understood she was in a phase of reproductive dormancy. As a result, her blood tests and ultrasounds were less than optimal, which her RE interpreted as POR. I encouraged her to have faith that her body and her ovaries had an ability to shift, and that she was not necessarily going into menopause.

Straight talk about stress

Because Chinese medicine is holistic, a TCM practitioner will ask about all aspects of your life, including how much stress you're dealing with, beyond the stress of trying to conceive. You probably think you're aware of your stress levels at work, at home, and in your life in general. But unless you are already employing effective stress-relieving strategies, any kind of stress—even good stress—can create imbalance and affect the environment you're creating for your unborn child.

In addition, women with fertility challenges may experience a very different type of stress. Please take a few minutes to ask yourself these questions and answer honestly to see how much of this stress you're enduring:

- When was the last time you laughed and had a good time?
- Are you avoiding friends and family?
- How many people know you're having some difficulty conceiving?
- Does your employer know you're trying to conceive? Do they offer any kind of support? What about your colleagues?

- Are you and your partner enjoying sexual intimacy or are you feeling pressured to perform?
- Do you avoid friends or family who are currently pregnant or have babies?
- Do you feel upset when you randomly see pregnant women or women with babies?
- Do you become upset if you see parents who you think are not responding to their child's needs as you think they should?
- Do you ask "Why them and not me?" or think "Everyone is getting pregnant except me?"
- Do you feel isolated and alone, thinking no one understands what you're going through?
- Have work and trying to conceive become your full-time jobs, or are you doing other things so they don't consume your life?

Unfortunately, when most women who come to my clinic answer these questions, they realize how isolated they feel and how consumed they've become with their fertility journey. Stress is part of living, but you can strategize to limit your stress where you can, create a supportive environment around yourself, seek ways to soften your reactions to stress, and make a positive difference in your own life.

Decreasing your stress levels

Acupuncture is one way to manage stress, but, realistically, you cannot do it every day. So what else can you do?

- Say "no." You do not have to agree to every request someone makes of you. Learn to say "no" to organizing a work event, going to a baby shower, or spending time with family or friends who do not support you.

- When you can't say "no," such as when your stress involves caring for a sick parent or grieving the loss of a loved one, acknowledge it. Close your eyes and notice where your stress is sitting in your body. Consciously relax that part of your body. Stress in and of itself does not impede pregnancy. It's how we respond to stress that may have a positive or negative impact on our body, mind, spirit, and ability to conceive.
- Connect with nature. Fresh air is healing. It can help you put things in perspective by seeing yourself as a small piece of the universe.
- Connect with your partner. Go for date nights. Keep intimacy alive. Remind yourselves why you became a couple.
- Go for walks. Moderate exercise helps work off stress hormones and replace them with feel-good hormones.
- Pick up a hobby. Find something you can be passionate about or something that just makes you smile, like pottery class, belly dancing, gardening, or crocheting.
- Create support. Talk to an understanding friend, join a fertility support group, or see a therapist who specializes in fertility. Do not rely on your partner's support, because there is a limit to how much he can support and understand you, especially when he is mourning in his own way, a way that is likely very different than yours. It is too much to ask any one person to fulfill every one of your physical, mental, and emotional needs. That's what friends and professionals are for.
- Assess whether you are a Type A personality, and realize you don't have to do it all and do it right. Every day, patients ask me "What else can I do?" I usually say, "What can you let go of today or this week?"
- Take the herbal medicines your TCM suggests. These are time-tested to allow for the free flow of energy throughout your body and nourish, restore, and replenish your energy, blood, body fluids, and essence.

- Try meditation or hypnosis. This does not have to be a sit-down thing, unless you have a personality that finds stillness rejuvenating. If you are a Type A, the exercises in the next bullet might be better for you.
- Try mind-body exercise like Tai Chi, Qi Gong, yoga, and even walking or running moderately. Any exercise that combines breathing with movement and increases self-awareness can have a calming, meditative effect on your body, mind, and spirit.
- Clean up your diet. Eating organic foods and minimizing your exposure to toxins can decrease the physical stress on your body.
- Practice gratitude. Create a routine when you wake up, before you go to bed, or before meals, where you think about one thing you are grateful for. Allow your mind to focus on one positive thing in your life, even if it's only for five minutes at a time. When I started working on this book, I created my social media Gratefulness Project, *365 Days of Keeping the Grass Greener on this Side,* to create a supportive environment for my readers and reduce my own worries. I find myself happier, more content, and less likely to sweat the small stuff. Practising gratitude can help you mitigate your stress as you deal with your fertility challenges.
- Learn to mother yourself first. When you are in an airplane with a child sitting beside you and the oxygen mask comes down, you put it on yourself first to ensure you'll be able to help your child. Mothering yourself means respecting and caring for yourself. In Avery's case, this meant understanding her own limitations and learning when to say "no" or ask for help. It meant going to work and doing her job well and then going home and leaving work behind. It meant taking yoga classes and going for walks with her husband, eating organic, hormone-free, pesticide-free, antibiotic-free

foods, and cutting out coffee and alcohol. And it meant recognizing how much to indulge her sweet tooth and when to stop.

- Remember, you are not your diagnosis. The fertility doctor's words made Avery feel broken, but she was not broken. She didn't need to feel imprisoned by her diagnosis, and neither do you. Instead, use your diagnosis as a jumping-off point, an opportunity to take care of yourself in ways you never have and see what happens.

The way TCM looks at your health

Avery reported herself to be healthy, active, and normal, with a regular menstrual cycle that was twenty-eight or twenty-nine days long. However, she experienced abdominal cramping and bloating, lower back pain, breast tenderness, lowered energy, and cravings for sweets for two days pre-menstrually and on the first day of her period. Even though these symptoms were normal for Avery, and typical for many women, they suggested an underlying imbalance as, according to TCM, menstruation should be uneventful and painless.

It's not unusual for a TCM practitioner to spend one-and-a-half to two hours with a patient on their first visit and sixty minutes on subsequent visits. This is not about running up fees but taking time to listen, question, counsel, provide lifestyle advice, check in on them emotionally and physically, provide dietary advice, suggest herbal medicine, and treat overall health, not just reproductive health, since everything is interrelated.

At each of our sessions, Avery was surprised at how much time I spent with her, especially when I was coming up with her TCM diagnosis. Women continue to be surprised by the questions I ask and the depth and precision of information I gather. In addition to asking about her overall health history, bodily functions, and lifestyle habits, TCM practitioners learn to diagnose illness by palpating the radial artery pulse and looking at the tongue.

When a TCM practitioner feels the radial artery through their finger pads, they are paying attention to the rate and rhythm of the pulse, as well as its qualities. How the blood flows within the blood vessels, and how fast it flows, indicates the person's health and vitality. Avery's pulse was deficient and slightly choppy.

To a TCM practitioner, the tongue provides another glimpse into the overall state of an individual's health. The tongue is the only visible internal muscle in the body. Its colour, size, and shape, as well as the thickness of the coating on it, reflect a lot about one's health. Avery's tongue was pale and swollen with teeth-marked edges, as if it was too big for her mouth. Increasing blood flow would make the tongue pinker, and increasing Qi (vital energy) would help the tongue hold its shape better.

To improve Avery's blood and energy flow, we began weekly acupuncture treatments and Chinese herbal medicines. She began to make some lifestyle changes, which included eating warm, cooked foods and drinking warm drinks, in contrast with her usual fare of frozen berry smoothies and cold salads. According to TCM, when we eat cold food and drink, we use energy to heat it before we can digest it. If we want as much energy as possible to go toward reproduction, we must conserve our energy by eating warm and easy-to-digest foods. Refer to Chapter 1 for more information on eating for fertility.

Preparing the soil for the seed

Avery liked the idea of preparing her body (soil) before she planted the seed. Her plan was that if she did not get pregnant naturally in six months, she would consider IVF. She was not interested in a donor egg from a young woman.

She changed her habits, going to sleep an hour earlier and sleeping eight hours each night. Soon she had more energy and was less irritable. She began using menstrual pads instead of tampons, as in TCM we believe menstrual blood is meant to flow out unimpeded rather than being plugged up, which can cause stagnation over time.

Within two months, Avery reported that her periods had become pain free for the first time in her life. When her period came, she would have a day of disappointment and sadness but, because she was feeling better overall, she felt more in control of her health. She wasn't focusing on her urgent need to be pregnant.

Feeling better physically allowed Avery to feel stronger emotionally, to process her feelings of sadness each month, often during our acupuncture sessions. Feeling better gave her hope that she was moving in the right direction by creating an internal environment that would welcome a child. She felt less desperate, more able to see what was possible rather than what her fertility doctor told her was not. As things improved, it made sense to work on her health for several months before trying IVF. After all, why plant the seed before the soil is ready?

Avery's welcome surprise

At one of her appointments, Avery came in panicked. "Mary, I think something is wrong. My period is six days late. I'm never late." I asked if she'd taken a pregnancy test and she said, "I've been putting it off because I don't think I could be pregnant. My husband had a business trip and we were only able to do it once, four days before ovulation."

I encouraged her to take the test. A week later, she announced her pregnancy with pride and joy and we altered our treatment strategy to support her pregnancy. She came in for treatments every week for the first trimester and monthly during her second trimester. At thirty-seven weeks, we resumed weekly treatments to help ripen Avery's cervix in preparation for a natural delivery. She went into labour twelve hours after our acupuncture treatment, just two days past her due date. Baby Alexander was born naturally six hours later, a healthy eight pounds, ten ounces.

3

More Than Surviving

Although you may not always be able to avoid
difficult situations, you can modify the extent to which you
can suffer by how you choose to respond to the situation.
DALAI LAMA XIV, *THE ART OF HAPPINESS*

Cary: Depression and antidepressants

Cary, a physician, was approaching forty-three and had been
trying to conceive for four years when her co-worker referred
her to me. She had attempted IVF twice, at forty and forty-one,
but her doctor had cancelled both attempts because the
injectable hormone drugs had failed to stimulate an increase
in egg production. On her third IVF attempt, her ovaries produced multiple follicles from which the doctor retrieved four
eggs, but although one was fertilized, no pregnancy resulted.

She came in devastated that her lifelong dream of having a
baby might never come true. She'd been with her first husband
since she was twenty, but when she was thirty-two and finally
ready to start a family, she caught him having an affair. More
stress followed as Cary's father divorced her mother, remarried,
and then fell ill and died. Overwhelmed by emotional trauma,
she began taking antidepressants and was still taking them
when she first came to see me.

"I really wanted to be in love with someone and have a baby," she told me. "So, I spent the next five years trying to find a partner, and didn't care about anything else." At thirty-eight, she met a man who wanted a baby, so they started trying. She loved him but didn't care whether it lasted; she just wanted a baby. But when she hit forty, she realized they were incompatible. Instead of looking for a new partner, she bought a house with a swing set in the back yard and a park beyond, and assumed she'd raise a child alone.

Ironically, the moment she stopped looking for true love, it landed on her doorstep. At forty, she married her next-door neighbour, ten years her senior. Without wasting time, they sought the help of a fertility clinic. Based strictly on her age, the doctor said there was no time to waste.

The RE diagnosed poor ovarian reserve (POR). Although her follicle stimulating hormone (FSH), a key indicator of ovarian aging, was still within normal limits, he said the shells of her eggs were hard. He doubted sperm would be able to penetrate her eggs naturally, so she'd probably need IVF with donor eggs. Adding insult to injury, he told her to lose weight, as if a clause in some contract dictated she wouldn't get pregnant unless she lost twenty pounds.

Like many of my patients, Cary came to me as a last resort, gravely disappointed that her life hadn't fallen into place as planned. But throughout this long journey, she'd opened herself to exploring every possible way to become a mother, through birth or otherwise. It was then that I told her about a previous patient with a similar fertility profile, including low ovarian reserve, who'd conceived through IUI without fertility medication.

The panic factor

When fertility doctors provide women with statistics and numbers showing they're reproductively old, even if they're only thirty-five, they don't intend to create panic, but this is often the effect. And if a woman is over forty and emotionally sensitive like Cary, they're likely to feel defective, depressed, and out of control.

The doctors' words cause women to fear they're in a race against time to conceive, but really those words represent an educated guess; no doctor knows for sure what's going to happen. For someone like Cary, who was anxious to begin with, the doctor's words exacerbated her emotional state. She tried to get off antidepressants but ended up staying on them and seeing a psychiatrist to help her manage her anxiety and depression.

Antidepressants and conception

A small amount of prescription medication for an adult is a huge amount for a tiny developing fetus. But what do you do when you have severe, unmanageable anxiety and depression, and nothing short of medication helps? The only right answer is the one that's right for you.

A 2015 study found that both continuous use of antidepressants and untreated major depression during pregnancy increase the incidence of premature delivery with all the potential accompanying health risks.[1] But if you have major depression, going off antidepressants may pose a greater risk for your mental and physical well-being than staying on them, and may put your baby at risk once you are pregnant.

Concerned about fetal health risks, Cary tried to get off antidepressants prior to trying to conceive but found medication was the only way to successfully manage her anxiety. Based on extensive advice from her psychiatrist, she stayed on a dose that was workable while she was trying to conceive.

If you wish to come off antidepressants, you must consult your doctor about the impacts on your mental and physical health. Whether you decide to wean yourself off medication (the only safe way to go off antidepressants), or you are trying to manage the stress and anxiety every woman feels when dealing with fertility challenges, there are things you can do to avoid panic, anxiety, and depression.

It can't be stressed enough

Based on my own experiences and those of the women and men I work with, dealing with the emotional and physical challenges of infertility on top of the ongoing stress of daily life can be difficult. For couples undergoing treatment at a fertility clinic, the drugs, daily appointments, and financial commitment add exponentially to the physical, emotional, and psychological burden.

One study showed that the stress women experience when trying to conceive is comparable to that of someone facing a life-threatening condition such as cancer.[2] Such stress triggers our bodies' fight-or-flight response. This instinctive reaction, which evolved millions of years ago to help us protect ourselves from perceived threats, diverts energy and blood flow to the heart, brain, and limbs so we can run away.

But modern-day stresses tend to be more chronic and overwhelming than the ones our bodies evolved to deal with. When our bodies stay in this protective mode constantly, we can feel chronically overwhelmed and anxious. The ongoing release of stress hormones can physically impede the ability to conceive, as there is little energy left over to reproduce when the body is focusing on survival.

One of the biggest stresses in dealing with fertility issues is the feeling of being out of control. In life generally, trying harder increases the likelihood that we will get what we're striving for. However, this does not work when it comes to baby-making. The harder you work at trying to conceive without success, and the more overwhelming and contradictory information you find, the more likely your stress levels will increase and your whole system will go into survival mode.

TCM can't reduce the stress in your life, but it can decrease your stress response by activating your *parasympathetic nervous system*, which controls the relaxation response in your body by slowing heart rate and relaxing blood vessels and muscles.[3] This can calm your nerves and help you change the way you think about your fertility, which can help you feel a little more in control of your life. It can help you feel like it's possible to thrive again rather than merely survive.

The effects of anxiety and depression

When you suppress your emotions and move through your life at a fast pace, you tend not to recognize stress building up over time like steam in a pressure cooker. You think this is just the way it is and push forward with your baby-making plan. At some point, seemingly out of nowhere, your pressure cooker will blow, and that's when you'll start experiencing anxiety and depression. To avoid that, you need to recognize the signs and symptoms of depression and find healthy outlets for your stress.

The following list of symptoms associated with depression was prepared for women undergoing fertility challenges by the American Society for Reproductive Medicine[4] and the Public Health Agency of Canada.[5] Are any of these signs familiar to you?

- Loss of interest in activities that brought joy in the past
- Depressed mood that doesn't lift
- Strained interpersonal relationships with partner, family, friends, and colleagues
- Difficulty thinking of anything other than your infertility
- High levels of anxiety
- Diminished ability to accomplish tasks
- Difficulty concentrating or making decisions

- Daytime tiredness
- Change in your sleep patterns (difficulty falling asleep or staying asleep, early morning awakening, or sleeping more than usual for you)
- Change in your appetite or weight (increase or decrease)
- Increased use of drugs or alcohol
- Persistent feelings of pessimism, guilt, worthlessness, help-lessness, or hopelessness
- Persistent feelings of bitterness or anger
- Decreased energy or fatigue (without significant physical exertion)
- Social isolation
- Thoughts about death or suicide

"Thrival skills" instead of survival skills

If you experience any of the above symptoms over a two-to-three-week period, please work with a registered mental health professional to get support. Don't ignore these symptoms; instead, acknowledge you're having challenges and be proactive. Having fertility challenges can lead to feeling out of control. This feeling can be triggered by going to a fertility clinic, seeing pregnant women all around you, or having someone tell you to "just relax." Please don't judge your own sensitivities, but try following my suggestions for developing "thrival skills" that can help you take back some control:

- Change your perspective. It always perplexes me when a doctor says a woman's eggs are old because it's more accurate to say the ovarian environment in which her eggs are growing is old. This is because your eggs start out as germ cells, which develop over 120 days. If you think of them as flowering seeds, TCM would tell you to nourish the soil before planting the seed so the plant will grow healthily.

- With that in mind, shift your focus and work on balancing your physical, mental, and emotional health so they will have a positive impact on the environment in which your eggs will develop over a three- or four-month period. Thinking this way can reduce the stress caused by a doctor telling you that you have "old eggs," and this can help maximize blood and energy flow to your ovaries and uterus, providing a more fertile environment for your developing eggs.
- FSH naturally increases and AMH and AFC naturally decrease as we age. This means your body might not respond well to fertility drugs. The drug used to stimulate egg growth is FSH, and if your body is already producing too much, adding more will not help. I equate it to trying to drive a car with your brakes on. Pushing the gas pedal (adding FSH) while your brakes are on (high FSH and decreasing AFC) will not help you drive the car.
- But having these indicators of lowered ovarian reserve does not mean you cannot get pregnant. It only means fertility drugs won't help. Gloria, whom we will read about in Chapter 4, became pregnant naturally despite her diagnoses of poor ovarian reserve, advanced maternal age, and secondary infertility. It makes me wonder how many women who have never set foot inside a fertility clinic conceive babies although they've never been tested and never know they had high FSH and low AMH at the time of conception.
- Acknowledge your feelings. An important aspect of avoiding or managing depression and anxiety is accepting and feeling your emotions as they happen, rather than harbouring them over prolonged periods. It's healthier to let feelings come and go like waves in the ocean, rather than bottling them up. When we fail to express negative emotions, they increase our stress levels, causing stress hormones to be released. This then launches us into the

fight-or-flight response, which interferes with our reproductive abilities.

- Create a community of support. Hang out with positive people or go out with friends you can confide in or just laugh with. Join a fertility support group if it suits you. Avoid negative people or environments. Do not watch upsetting news.

- Meditate and breathe. Meditation and breathing help to calm your mind and make you feel connected to your body. Close your eyes and sit or lie down in a comfortable position as you focus on your breath. Count to four slowly upon inhalation and then count to eight upon exhalation. This will give your brain a little break, even if it's only for five minutes at a time to pull yourself out of the fight-or-flight mode. This activates your parasympathetic nervous system, which enhances hormone production.[6]

- Visualize. This can be a form of meditation that creates a calming response, especially if you close your eyes and picture a place you associate with peace, calm, and tranquility. It might be your favourite vacation spot, or any other place you dream of being, like a rain forest, by the ocean, up a mountain, or in front of a cozy fire.

- Exercise. Exercise not only releases endorphins, which enhance mood, but also gets you out of your head and more connected to your body. Choose something you like; don't force yourself to do something you hate just because it's supposed to be good for you. If you don't know what to choose, try different activities, like yoga, walking, Tai Chi, Qi Gong, dancing, paddle boarding, golfing, tennis, swimming—anything that gets you moving, but gently. Avoid adrenaline sports!

- Live a little. Instead of devoting every waking thought to getting pregnant, do things that make you laugh and have fun and feel fulfilled. You could take up a new hobby or revisit something you have enjoyed in the past, such as salsa dancing, singing Karaoke, playing an instrument, writing, painting, going out with friends, or gardening.

- Eat whole foods. When you are depressed, you might have symptoms like daytime tiredness, difficulties accomplishing tasks, and high levels of anxiety. This can make it difficult to cook or source out healthy foods, yet good food will help you feel better. Eating whole organic foods without preservatives helps you nourish your body and prevent nutritional deficiencies that may contribute to depression and poor physical health.

- Take supplements. Consult a nutritionist or naturopathic doctor to assess whether nutritional deficiencies might be contributing to your depression. These deficiencies can include:

  > Vitamin D, 3000 IU per day.[7]

  > Folate, one gram per day. In addition to being good for pregnancy, folate increases the therapeutic effects of antidepressants.[8]

  > Vitamin B12, but it is better to increase intake through foods such as eggs, poultry, fish, and lean meats, as supplements can interact with antidepressant drugs.[9]

  > Omega-3 fatty acids, 3000 mg (2500 mg EPA/500 mg DHA).[10]

  > L-tryptophan, an essential amino acid found in beef, turkey, cottage cheese, and almonds, which converts to and increases levels of serotonin, a natural mood lifter. It can also be taken as 5HTP, 200 mg per day.[11]

- Get acupuncture and TCM. TCM, which incorporates acupuncture, Chinese herbal medicine, and lifestyle counselling, has been used to treat and prevent depression for thousands of years in China. Acupuncture and Chinese medicine have been researched and shown to improve depression. One study stated weekly acupuncture for three months significantly reduced symptoms of depression compared to antidepressant medication alone, and acupuncture was similarly effective to counselling.[12]

- Chinese herbs are prescribed according to an individual's presentation of symptoms. That means that we cannot give the same herbal formula for every case of depression. Despite that, numerous trials have shown combining different Chinese herbs with antidepressants to be more effective in treating depression than antidepressants alone.[13]

Review the lists on page 40 of Chapter 2 on decreasing your stress levels and page 52 of Chapter 4 for additional tips on how to change your survival skills to "thrival" skills.

Focusing on energy instead of eggs

In TCM, we believe you are born with a certain amount of energy inherited from your parents. The process of digestion and transportation of food and drink throughout your body provides a source for Gu Qi, or nutritive energy, that feeds all the cells in your body. When something disrupts or weakens this process, less energy is available to support your well-being. This can create imbalances, which can lead to depression or fertility challenges. So as part of preparing the soil, you need to look not only at what you eat but how you eat (Refer to Chapter 1, Eating for fertility: How and when to eat.)

Kidney tapping and rubbing

In Chinese medicine, the kidney energy is the foundation of all of the other internal organs, including the reproductive organs. Invigorating and nourishing the kidneys is therefore fundamental to your fertile health. Coincidentally, nerve innervations to the ovaries and uterus are located between the vertebrae from thoracic 12 (mid-back) to the sacrum (lower back).

1. Stand with your feet hip-width apart, toes pointed outward at 45 degrees.
2. Keep your knees soft.
3. Place the back of your hands along your back in the kidney areas (from the bottom of your ribs to your waist and sacrum, or T12–L3 and L3–S4). Rub up and down for two to three minutes, until the area feels warm.
4. With cupped hands (thumb and index finger together), lightly tap the kidney area, alternating on the left and right sides. This should feel soothing and not uncomfortable.

I watched my grandmother do this every morning to invigorate her organs. She lived to the ripe old age of ninety-four.

How Cary learned to thrive

Cary admitted that she hadn't thought paying close attention to all aspects of her health could make a difference to her fertility, but she was willing to try. She'd invested four years in IVF treatments and she'd never been told to change any aspects of her health routines. She eagerly started pre-conception treatments with me for four months. This included lifestyle changes, supplementation, and some emotional release work:

- She began biking to and from work, jogging twice a week, and doing yoga, which helped work off some of the stress. In TCM, we say mild exercise and meditative movements can de-stagnate energy that gets built up and congested over time.

- She attended a mindfulness meditation course, which taught her to be still, present, and true to herself moment by moment.
- She changed her dietary habits by buying organic fruits, vegetables, and meats as much as possible, and cutting down her intake of fast foods by seventy-five percent, which felt better in general as she had more energy and felt less bloated.
- She took Royal Jelly (the food reserved for the queen bee, which produces all the worker bees in the colony) and Ubiquinol (see Chapter 4). She felt mentally clearer and more energetic.
- She joined a fertility support group, which helped her deal with the emotional consequences of her fertility challenges.
- She and her husband had sex regularly, without watching the calendar, and surrendered to the process. Each month she did not conceive, her tears for the loss of a potential baby had the effect of a physical, emotional, and spiritual cleanse.
- We did weekly acupuncture treatments for four months to support Cary's emotional healing.

More than a physical treatment

Cary was grief-stricken by the combination of her first love's infidelity, her parents' divorce, her father's death, and her inability to conceive. The accumulated emotional trauma consumed her and tied up her energy. Over time, this led to other imbalances, with symptoms including menstrual pain, severe low back pain, extreme exhaustion, anxiety, and increased susceptibility to stress.

As often happens with my patients, when I inserted acupuncture needles into different points along the body, Cary's physical pains were relieved. But even more important for her healing, she was able to tap into and release the intense grief she held deep inside her body, which she couldn't get out by herself. Cary said that during the acupuncture treatments she went through an exploration process and accepted that her pregnancy was not happening naturally, and she processed her grief and losses. She said that all of these layers of healing happened at the same time, guided by the treatments.

I remember Cary crying every time she had a treatment—and it wasn't because the needles were hurting her. As her body relaxed with each treatment, tears would stream down her face in a much-needed release of emotions locked deep within her physical body. I remember the first time this happened, she said, "I don't know why, but I feel like crying." Afterwards, her mood lifted as the acupuncture allowed her to access her grief, which remained a pervasive undercurrent in her body, and little by little, she moved along her pathway to healing.

Not everyone cries and experiences a physical emotional release through acupuncture, but most women walk away feeling more relaxed, less stressed, and more ready to face whatever lies ahead. It is a safe way to precipitate a release of emotional energy that gets trapped over time.

Cary thanked me for giving her a safe space to cry and for connecting with her in a way she had been unable to connect with other practitioners. The fact that I fully understood her pain and despair comforted her and gave her hope. Her release enabled her to find her own voice, trusting that the answers to her problems might be found outside the medical model.

The impact of IVF drugs on body and mind

Although I didn't treat Cary specifically for the side effects of IVF drugs, they could easily have contributed to her pre-existing anxiety and depression. Just making the decision to try IVF can be stressful. It's not something you'd ever dream of going through when you were a little girl. Yet millions of women undergo IVF every year and not everyone gets pregnant.

One 2015 study in the UK found that the live-birth rate for the first cycle of IVF was less than thirty percent out of 156,947 women where the average age was between thirty-two and thirty-eight.[14] Clearly, IVF is not a magic bullet. Some women conceive the first time they try IUI or IVF, but many do not. Some fertility doctors even say your chances of a successful pregnancy are based on six rounds of IVF, not one.[15] If you choose IVF, you need to have realistic expectations about your chances of conceiving, as well as the potential for side effects.

Because I see women on IVF drugs every day, I routinely ask them to report side effects. Thankfully, they are not long term, as the drugs leave the system within days to months. But each woman is as unique as her experiences, and the following possible symptoms may vary greatly from mild to severe:

- Headaches
- Hives
- Local pain
- Ovarian hyper-stimulation
- Abdominal bloating
- Constipation
- Hot flashes, night sweats, dizziness (more like full-on menopausal symptoms)
- Insomnia
- Vivid dreams
- Nausea
- Tiredness
- Breast tenderness and distension

In addition, there can be mood swings, from depression and sadness to irritability, anxiety, and anger (these may all be present due to the stress of infertility itself, but the fertility drugs heighten them dramatically). If you've been using injectable hormones, there can be pain, redness, and swelling at the needle site. And if you've been using progesterone vaginal suppositories, there can be itching or yeast infections. (When yeast infections occur, I recommend putting suppositories up the rectum. It doesn't sound like a great option, but when you are suffering from a yeast infection, the "back end" doesn't sound so bad.)

Every woman responds differently to fertility drugs; some tell me they experience no side effects, while others experience many of the above symptoms. There are oral and injectable drugs; some women respond horribly to oral and better to injectable, while for some it's the other way around.

Minimizing side effects

Every day in my clinic I help women minimize the effects of their fertility treatments. If you are thinking of getting help from a fertility clinic, please also consider finding a TCM practitioner who can provide the kind of support I give my patients. This typically includes:

- Acupuncture, which has been well documented for treating pain of any kind.[16, 17] It helps by reducing stress[18] as one goes through IVF. I use acupuncture every day with my patients to alleviate many of the drug side effects listed above.
- Chinese herbs, which vary depending on your symptoms. You must consult a TCM practitioner to treat and support your body and specific symptoms as you go through hormonal treatments. Although herbal medicine is still not widely used in North America, TCM is widely used in China and has been clinically shown to be beneficial and increase pregnancy rates. In a study done by Lee Hullender Rubin, when acupuncture and other TCM modalities were used

before and in conjunction with IVF medical treatment, the TCM group produced thirteen percent more live births than the group that received IVF alone.[19]

Be aware that your reproductive endocrinologist (RE) may disapprove of your use of TCM, if he or she has not studied the use of Chinese herbs. When doctors don't know about herbal medicine, they fear negative interactions with fertility drugs, as well as potential toxicity from the herbs.

Doctors' concerns notwithstanding, many women take herbal medicine leading up to IVF. A greater number take herbal medicines prior to IUI, partly because there are fewer drugs involved, but also because IUI is less costly than IVF, so there is less fear of drug interactions interfering with the success of the procedure. However, some women who have had previous negative results with IVF feel they have nothing to lose by adding Chinese medicine.

Like acupuncture, the aim of Chinese herbal medicine is to help restore balance in the body in order to optimize overall health, as well as the health of the eggs, sperm, and uterus. In China, it's commonplace to use drugs and Chinese herbs simultaneously. The drugs and herbs do different things, and there is no reason to fear negative drug interactions when you see a qualified TCM doctor. However, if you are at a fertility clinic, you need to feel comfortable working with your RE. So, if your RE is adamant about not using Chinese herbs, you may choose to comply.

Cleansing from fertility drugs

Thankfully, whether the hormones are taken orally, through injections, or by suppository, the body naturally eliminates them after several months. After my failed IVF cycles, I did a liver cleanse to eliminate the hormonal drugs before going on to the next cycle, to ensure the drug response would be optimal each time. I ate cruciferous vegetables, such as cabbage and broccoli,[20] and took supplements, such as milk thistle[21] and wheatgrass, so that my body would bounce back for the next IVF cycle.

Cary's last intervention

After four months of pre-conception treatment, Cary decided to do one last round of IUI. Her fertility doctor discouraged her, telling her not to waste her money and reiterating that her eggs were old and impenetrable. He didn't think artificial insemination would help fertilization.

Cary practiced her mindfulness techniques and her visualization exercises, releasing the doctor's negative words and instead focusing on appreciating the work she'd done during the previous four months. Even though her doctor didn't think Cary had a chance of getting pregnant, he humoured her and went forward with an IUI protocol.

First, he prescribed a five-day course of Clomid, an oral fertility drug. Instead of making multiple eggs, as hoped, Cary grew just one egg. To make sure she ovulated, the doctor injected her with Ovidril, a drug known to help ripen the developing egg and trigger ovulation. Cary also continued with her acupuncture treatments to help prepare the soil before planting the seed.

Even though she hadn't lost those twenty pounds the doctor had recommended, she had been taking great care of herself physically and emotionally. As a TCM practitioner, I believe that was enough to allow the miracle of life to flow through her and she became pregnant by combining the help of both Eastern and Western medicine. On her doctor's advice, she stayed on antidepressants to help stabilize her depression and prevent anxiety during her pregnancy, which left untreated could have posed risks both to the baby's neurological development and in the form of premature labour and delivery.[22] Nine months later, she gave birth to Brandon, a healthy baby boy.

Cary's story reminds us to look at our age and diagnosis as a baseline from which to explore other options. Rather than letting age limit us, which can consume us and cause grave despair, we can focus on aligning ourselves harmoniously in body, mind, and spirit. We are unique individuals, and sometimes, the creation of life transcends numbers and statistics. Science can support the creation of a baby, but it can't dictate when the miracle of life happens.

4

Doing More Is Not Always Doing Better

The secret of health for both mind and body is not to
mourn for the past, worry about the future, or anticipate troubles,
but to live in the present moment wisely and earnestly.

BUDDHA

Gloria: Secondary infertility

At thirty-nine years old, it hit Gloria for the first time that she
wanted to have a child. She'd been on the birth control pill since
she was seventeen. Two months after she came off it, she conceived her first child on their first try, giving birth to George at
the age of forty. Overjoyed with creating a family, Gloria and
her husband started to try for a second child when George was
two. It took her six months to get pregnant, but she miscarried
at five weeks. She was crushed, especially after it had been so
easy getting pregnant with George.

We cannot underestimate the drive to have a baby, even for
a woman who already has one. Once a couple has a child, they
often feel obligated to provide a sibling. Parents who have
difficulty often feel guilty and inadequate. Their guilt is often
compounded by their knowledge that many women and

couples struggling with fertility do not have a child at all. They feel ungrateful, and sometimes sense these women are judging them.

Having difficulty conceiving after already having given birth is a struggle for many women. The hope of having a second child carries as much anticipation and longing as it does for a woman hoping to become pregnant for the first time. If this difficulty is followed by miscarriage, it can also bring additional stress and worry, rather than joy, during the early months after the woman finally conceives.

What is secondary infertility?

I have seen and helped many women who had difficulties conceiving a second child. This is called *secondary infertility*. After the miscarriage, concerned about her age (now forty-three), Gloria met with a fertility doctor who discouraged her from trying IVF.

Gloria was in the advanced maternal age category. As seen on day three of her menstrual cycle, Gloria didn't have many antral follicles, which is normal for a woman of her age. Because of that, IVF was not her best option. The doctor assured her that it didn't mean she couldn't have a baby; it just meant the methods they'd normally use to assist pregnancy were not going to help.

I was pleased that Gloria's RE acknowledged that her age didn't mean she couldn't have a baby. In TCM, we see birth and delivery as among the most energy-draining experiences in a woman's life. In terms of Jing Qi, our primordial energy, endowed at birth through our parents, gets depleted as we live our lives. Birthing drains a lot of it.

Gloria's doctor's recommendations came from the United States Government's Centers for Disease Control (CDC) Assisted Reproductive Technology National Summary Report.[1] Statistically speaking, women over forty-three using IVF have a less than five percent chance of having a baby through IVF, compared to women under thirty-five, who have up to a sixty percent chance of having a live birth after IVF.

That makes IVF an expensive endeavour. The drugs used for IVF can only stimulate the growth of the eggs that are there at the beginning of each menstrual cycle. At forty-three, if only two or three *antral follicles* (AF) are visible on the third day of your menstrual cycle, that is the maximum number of follicles that can potentially grow to maturity and be surgically retrieved at ovulation. A woman under thirty-five typically has at least double that amount. The fewer follicles retrieved, the fewer eggs become fertilized, and the lower the chances of making a baby.

My view on IVF statistics and numbers

I do not dispute the fact that the number of antral follicles that could potentially grow to mature eggs when stimulated by hormonal drugs decreases with age. IVF does not make sense if your *antral follicle count* (AFC) will only increase your chances of pregnancy by five percent or less. That said, I have seen some women older than forty with AFCs like that of a thirty-year-old (that is, instead of a vaginal ultrasound showing four follicles at the beginning of the menstrual cycle, it shows twelve). If that is the case, IVF is not a bad option.

However, the fact that IVF is not always the right choice does not mean a woman over thirty-five cannot get pregnant naturally. We are all unique and what works for one person may not work for another. Instead of looking at technology as the only option, an older woman might consider other, more natural ways to optimize her reproductive health, which I will share later in this chapter.

How TCM views aging

As we age, our energy levels decrease. You can probably relate to this: you no longer party into the wee hours of the morning and go to work afterwards, as you may have done in your youth. In your late thirties or early forties, you may feel exhausted even thinking about an all-nighter!

In Chinese medicine, we recognize this as our life force energy, Qi. As mentioned earlier, in TCM, we believe we are born with a certain amount of energy. I equate this to gas in a car. Typically, we are born with a full tank of gas, which we use up as we move through life. In terms of fertility, we have a certain amount of energy to develop eggs each cycle. As we age, our energy naturally declines, which leads to fewer eggs that can potentially grow in each cycle, known as a lowered AFC.

But regardless of your age, and no matter how many eggs are available in each cycle, you typically develop one egg (or sometimes two) to maturity at ovulation. If you use hormonal medications to develop all the eggs available in a cycle, there will be a lower yield for a woman of forty-three years than for a thirty-year-old. In my view, if you are forty-three, it's more efficient to harness the energy you have to focus naturally on that one leading follicle, rather than trying to divide your energy in the hope of developing more than one egg through medication.

In this case, having more eggs does not increase chance of pregnancy; it may even do the opposite. There are ways to conserve and enhance your energy so it can go toward egg production. Because your body, mind, and spirit require energy to function, you must be mindful of how you use your energy and careful not to waste it. What you eat and drink, how you live your life, how you avoid and manage stress—all of this has an impact on your energy and may affect your ability to conceive.

Don't do more—do better

When women and couples have difficulty conceiving, many assume that doing more (technology and drugs) will get them pregnant faster. This is not true, especially in the case of a mature woman with a reduced AFC. But that doesn't mean you cannot conceive.

You might think, "More is more," but by doing more, you might become less balanced. As interventions become increasingly intrusive, the process of making a baby becomes more physically and emotionally demanding. Just going to the fertility clinic for daily blood work and ultrasounds on top of your already busy life can increase your stress levels. The drugs can have energy-draining side effects, and the more drugs you take, the greater your chances of having side effects. All of this creates imbalance that potentially takes you further away from your natural ability to conceive.

This was the case for Gloria. She wanted to get pregnant as soon as possible and thought IVF was the answer. Despite the advice from the fertility doctor not to do IVF, she attempted four cycles of IVF (two cycles of which were downgraded to IUI due to a lack of response) back to back, all without achieving pregnancy.

The lack of response made her feel empty, so instead of pursuing more fertility treatments, she went to see a naturopathic doctor and started taking supplements. She looked into acupuncture and met me for the first time one month after her last failed IVF. After five months of taking supplements and doing acupuncture weekly, she became pregnant naturally—but she miscarried.

There was nothing I could say that could make that better. Miscarriage hurts; I know because I have been there myself. I told her I was sorry for her sadness and grief, but it was important to allow herself to go through it. I said I strongly believed her body knew how to be pregnant, as she'd already proven with George. I told her I couldn't guarantee anything and didn't know how long she would be willing to continue her journey to conceive, but that I did think it was possible for her to conceive a healthy baby and carry it to term.

Gloria decided to continue pursuing the natural route to pregnancy and told me she was willing to keep trying until she was forty-nine. She planned to continue TCM, acupuncture, and supplements to decrease her stress, maintain balance, and optimize the quality of her eggs. She subsequently became pregnant and miscarried a third time about a year later, at forty-four.

Finally, a month after she turned forty-five, her patience, perseverance, and persistence (what I call the 3 Ps) paid off when she conceived Dylan. In retrospect, she said she felt the stress of IVF, including the impact of the hormonal drugs and the demands of going to the clinic daily, while juggling childcare and work, actually impeded her ability to get pregnant.

Boosting fertility naturally

When I asked Gloria why she thought she was successful in having a baby, she replied, "I think a combination of everything I did led me to have Dylan. It could have been the supplements or the acupuncture. The one thing I find interesting is that the month I got pregnant you told me to just relax and maybe think about donors. And that's what I was doing. I was thinking about how best to convince my husband to go through donor eggs from a young person. I researched potential donors I found online through an agency and made a whole list of the donors I liked and then—boom!—I was pregnant."

Here's what Gloria did:

- She and her husband had sex daily from after her period until after ovulation (not everyone can do this without feeling too stressed to perform).
- Because she had a family, she did not follow a specific fertility diet, but she:
  > Ate mostly organic, home-cooked meals.
  > Avoided junk food.

- > Ate whole wheat, spelt, or whole-grain pasta, bread, and crackers (her husband was half Italian and they ate a lot of carbs, so she was not willing to give them up).
- > Drank two cups of organic coffee every morning without worrying about caffeine's negative consequences. (Gloria felt that, for her, the benefits of feeling alert in the morning outweighed the risk of miscarriage.)
- She had acupuncture treatments weekly for most of two years before conceiving Dylan, and kept it up during her pregnancy to maximize blood flow to her uterus and increase her relaxation response.
- She took supplements, including:
  - > Royal Jelly, one capsule three times daily (see Chapter 3) to boost her energy.
  - > PQQ (Pyrroloquinoline quinone) 10 mg daily, and Ubiquinol 400 mg (200 mg twice daily). Ubiquinol is the metabolized form of Coenzyme Q10 (CoQ10), which occurs naturally in the body. It is known in both Eastern and Western medicine as a powerful antioxidant that supplies energy to cells. Because there is a natural decline of energy in the cells (including eggs) as we age, PQQ (another powerful antioxidant) and Ubiquinol can help increase cellular energy to aid proper cell division, which can potentially decrease chromosomal abnormalities associated with aging.
  - > MTHF (methylfolate), one gram. MTHF is more readily absorbable than folic acid, which is essential to fetal development.
  - > Prenatal multivitamins.

Most importantly, toward the end she stopped trying to force a baby into her belly. Until then, she had been obsessive. It was when she shifted her focus to finding a potential egg donor that she became pregnant. From a TCM perspective, I feel that when she stopped obsessing, her stress levels decreased and her subsequent relaxation response increased the energy available to her womb. And like magic, baby Dylan came to be.

Obsessing doesn't help

When Gloria and many of the women I encounter try to have a baby, they obsess about it, putting a lot of pressure on themselves to succeed. In terms of Chinese medical theory, this kind of obsession consumes energy. If we have a limited amount of energy in our bodies, when we consume energy through excessive thinking, worries, and fears, we have less energy available for conception. These worries and fears may cause enough stress to create a fight-or-flight response (see Chapter 3), which diverts energy away from the reproductive organs to where it is needed most for survival (the brain, heart, and limbs).

Miscarriage facts

Fertility challenges, including miscarriages, are the most common pregnancy complication, occurring in fifteen to twenty-five percent of all pregnancies. Approximately five percent of couples will experience two consecutive losses, and one percent will experience three or more first-trimester miscarriages.[2] The miscarriage rate in women under thirty-five is between eight and twelve percent; it climbs as high as forty-five percent in those over forty.[3]

The rates may be even higher. Because miscarriage is a private subject, many women and couples experience it behind closed doors and do not tell people about it. Only in recent years did I discover that my mother, who married at sixteen, had a miscarriage before she conceived my brother at seventeen and me at nineteen. I had two miscarriages before conceiving Zoe.

Mark Zuckerberg, founder and CEO of Facebook, reported that he and his wife, Priscilla Chan, had three miscarriages over several years when they were in their late twenties. As one of the world's most influential people, I was deeply moved by his courage and openness in talking about their recurrent losses when announcing their pregnancy on July 31, 2015, on Facebook. When a person of Zuckerberg's influence speaks publicly about fertility challenges, it goes a long way to reducing stigma and ignorance around these issues.

Not all miscarriages are alike

Although medical science would like to say Gloria's miscarriages were likely the result of advanced maternal age and egg quality issues, we know that in the medical model many factors can lead to miscarriage.[4] These can include:

- Chromosomal abnormalities.
- Birth defects, which can impede the implantation and growth of a fetus. These can include uterine anomalies like a *septate uterus* (where a septum, or wall, divides the uterus in two); *uterine fibroids* (abnormal growths in the uterus); an *incompetent (open) cervix* (the cervix is normally closed during pregnancy; if it is open, it may not retain a pregnancy); endometrial polyps (the *endometrium* is the inner mucous membrane of the uterus); and *Asherman's syndrome* (uterine scarring).
- Autoimmune issues or immunologic disorders, such as *thrombophilia* (a blood-clotting issue), or another condition in which the body attacks the sperm or embryo as if it were a foreign invader.
- *Polycystic ovarian syndrome* (PCOS), a hormonal imbalance causing the ovaries to make more androgens than normal, which interferes with the development and release of eggs.

- Clinical or sub-clinical thyroid disorders. Thyroid stimulating hormone (TSH) levels even at the low end of what's medically considered normal for most people increases risk of miscarriage by sixty-nine percent because of the increased demand pregnancy puts on your thyroid.[5]
- Diabetes, which can lead to ovulation disorders and tubal blockage.[6]
- Bacterial infections.
- Lifestyle factors, including exposure to:
  > Alcohol and drugs.
  > Environmental toxins like *xenoestrogens* (endocrine disruptors with estrogen-like effects), which may be found in chemicals and pesticides and which can affect hormones.
  > *Phthalates*, an ingredient found in soft plastic bags (for food and even plastic bags for blood transfusions or IVS), cosmetics, hair care products, cologne, aftershave, shampoo, nail polish, hair spray, and some time-release medications.[7]
  > *Bisphenol-A* (BPA), found in plastics and in the linings of cans, which can exhibit hormonal properties not safe for pregnancy and has been shown to cause chromosomal abnormalities in the eggs of mice.[8]
  > Heavy metals like lead and mercury, which have been linked not only to miscarriage, but to impotence, decreased fertility in women, lowered sperm counts, and decreased libido in men.[9]

Although the long list of things that can go wrong with pregnancy may make you wonder how anyone gets pregnant at all, the case studies in this book provide living proof that miracles do happen despite these diagnoses.

Barbara: Recurrent miscarriages

Barbara, who was a decade younger than Gloria, also had recurrent miscarriages, although she had a very different health history. I met Barbara when she was thirty-one. She and her husband had been trying to conceive for two and a half years. She had miscarried twice before going to her family physician to get blood work and a *sonohysterogram*, a test where a salt-water solution is injected into the uterus, which is then viewed through ultrasound to expose abnormalities that might contribute to miscarriage. Although the procedure was painful, it showed nothing that accounted for her miscarriages.

Barbara's family doctor then prescribed Clomid, an oral fertility drug, for five days early in her menstrual cycle to increase the number of follicles she would ovulate. She experienced nausea, bloating, irritability, hot flashes, and weight gain. She did not conceive the first two times. On her third cycle, she conceived but miscarried at six weeks. Frustrated and deeply saddened, she decided to take a break.

Even though no physical factors (by Western medical standards) accounted for Barbara's recurrent miscarriages, she knew intuitively that she was feeling "off" physically and emotionally. She feared she could not handle another loss and wanted to look for a more natural approach that would help her feel whole again. It is not unusual for women who have experienced recurrent miscarriages to feel as if a little of them dies each time one of their potential babies dies.

Signs of imbalance

Thousands of years before modern assisted reproductive technology was developed, Chinese medicine recognized that the body gives us signs of imbalance. The art of feeling how the blood flows within the blood vessels is an indicator of health or imbalance. Barbara's pulse felt strong underneath my fingertips but bound and tense like a guitar string rather than free-flowing like a stream. This indicated stress in her body, so I asked her about it. She confirmed that, over the past three years, she'd experienced several traumatic events. Her mother had died of breast cancer, and in the final stages, Barbara had spent weekends nursing her. Six months after her mother passed on, her dog, who had been with her family for twelve years, had to be put down. And now, she and her husband were dealing with his father recovering from surgery for prostate cancer.

As Barbara reflected on her previous few years, she could see why her body was in survival mode, rather than baby-making mode. Through my clinical experience, I have seen how stress-related anxiety and depression over prolonged periods can impede fertility. Emotional stress can cause heightened levels of *cortisol*, a stress hormone that may impede the brain's ability to produce the proper cascade of reproductive hormones necessary to produce a healthy egg, develop the uterine lining, and grow a fertilized egg into an embryo. From a TCM perspective, if we have a finite amount of energy, and most of it is consumed by stresses such as dealing with death and dying, including repeated miscarriage, there is less energy available to create the spark of life and keep it going.

You don't have to be stress-free in order to get pregnant and have a healthy baby, but the way you handle your stress can have a positive or negative impact on your health and well-being, overall and reproductively. Barbara was a private and quiet person. She had been bottling up her emotions for years while caring for everyone around her. I encouraged her to find ways to decrease the impact of stress in her life and develop skills to relieve her stress for when she did become pregnant. Upon my recommendation, she joined a fertility support group and connected with women who fully understood her feelings.

Decreasing the impact of stress during pregnancy

Here are some things you can engage in and practice to soften the impact of stress in your life while you are pregnant:

- Keep yourself in a happy bubble. Find a little laughter by reading funny books or magazines, watching funny movies, or hanging out with good friends. Laughter increases the relaxation response and may lighten your stress load during pregnancy. Stay away from bad news.[10]
- Sleep. Rest is very important. If you're exhausted, don't force yourself to exercise, since you need most of your energy to create a baby. Give yourself permission to nap, rest, and not overwork. Decrease your stress levels by conserving your energy.
- Connect with people you love. Plan date nights with your partner (even if they're in the comfort of your own home when you are tired and pregnant). Have a phone date or in-person visit with a friend or family member who comforts and supports you.
- Go for acupuncture. Acupuncture has been used for thousands of years to help pregnant women reduce stress and increase blood flow to the womb.
- Limit yourself to thirty minutes or an hour per day of research on your electronic device. Knowing more about the world can cause you more stress. And typically, the more you read, the more contradictory information you will find, which can cause you even more stress.

Also review the list on decreasing your stress levels on page 40 of Chapter 2 and the list of "thrival skills" on page 52 of Chapter 3.

Meditative breathing and visualization

In addition to following the tips offered on the previous page for decreasing the impact of stress during pregnancy, practice meditative breathing and visualization. First, close your eyes and take a deep breath. Allow your thoughts to come and go. Do not suppress anything. Acknowledge that they are just thoughts and not statements of fact.

Notice where you feel these thoughts in your body. That is, where do you feel the tension in your body as these negative thoughts come up, and what does it feel like? Is it a knot in the stomach, or tension in the neck, shoulders, or jaws? Stay with the sensation and notice if you see a colour associated with it. Does it have a temperature? Is it associated with an emotion? What is it saying to you?

Be with your body. Notice whether the sensations, colours, and feelings change as you focus on your body. As you inhale, feel the knot or tension and visualize yourself directing oxygen to that part of the your body; as you exhale, invite that part of your body to release and expel the tension with the outgoing breath. Move your body slightly to a position that feels most comfortable for the tension. Allow it to dissipate, melt away, or move down and out of the body with every breath. Notice your whole body and allow it to relax. Shift your legs and your hands to a more relaxed position. After you feel relaxed, come back to an awareness of your surroundings. Stretch your arms and legs and, when you are ready, open your eyes and go on with your day.

Navigating neuroses in early pregnancy

You endure the two-week wait and find out you are pregnant at last. You should be celebrating, but instead you find yourself waiting in dread for another miscarriage. When you read online or go to a fertility clinic, where the focus is pathology, it's difficult to fully embrace your pregnancy. You are anxious and keep looking for pregnancy symptoms to reassure yourself that you are still pregnant. Barbara did it. Gloria did it. I did it as well.

Every woman experiences pregnancy differently. Some feel symptom-free throughout the first trimester; others experience symptoms on and off but develop more symptoms later. My goal here is to shed some light on what to expect in early pregnancy, in the hope of decreasing your stress levels and increasing your relaxation response to help optimize the health of your developing baby.

Here are some of the most common signs of early pregnancy. But if you don't have them, don't panic; your pregnancy may still be perfectly normal:

- Fatigue. This is the most common pregnancy sign I see in my clinic. You may find yourself exhausted and dragging your feet all day, caused by a rise in progesterone levels. This simply means your body is hard at work building nutrient- and oxygen-rich blood vessels in your uterine lining to support your growing baby through the first twelve weeks of pregnancy, and simultaneously getting a placenta ready for second trimester.

  If you're tired, give yourself permission to nap when you can. Think of it as your body's way of telling you to slow down, conserve your energy, and allow your system to focus on your womb. If you tended to be anemic or iron deficient before pregnancy, take a prenatal supplement with iron; you need iron to make the hemoglobin found in red blood cells, which carries oxygen. In pregnancy, your blood volume doubles, resulting in an increased demand for iron and oxygen. If you become deficient, your fatigue will increase.
- Breast tenderness. If you suspect you're pregnant, you likely feel your breasts every chance you get to make sure they're still tender and swollen. You might even freak out

if they aren't tender. Just remind yourself the next time you cop a feel that it's normal for breast tenderness to be inter-mittent or absent during early pregnancy. You have nine months, lots of time for your breasts to grow and produce milk for your baby.

- Morning sickness. You hear about women complaining of nausea and vomiting during their first trimester. In my practice, most women worry if they are not nauseous. Some women have no nausea at all while others feel it come and go throughout the day. Nausea can be aggravated by not eating regularly, eating too much in one sitting, or feeling tired. Acupuncture works well to treat it—sometimes a little too well. I've had women return a week after a treatment requesting that I do not take away their nausea completely because it reassures them they're still pregnant!

Other normal symptoms of early pregnancy may include:

- Increased emotional sensitivity
- Heightened sense of smell
- Cravings or aversions to specific foods
- Increased urinary frequency
- Changes in libido
- Shortness of breath
- Twinges in the lower abdomen

Being monitored at the fertility clinic

If you've been pregnant before and are using a fertility clinic, your doctor may want to monitor you more frequently than a woman who hasn't had challenges conceiving. For me, this was a blessing and a curse—a blessing because I got to see my baby developing, but a curse because the more tests I had, the more I worried about each test in advance.

When I was pregnant with Zoe, I had to go for blood tests every other day for ten days. The doctor wanted to make sure my *beta HCG* was doubling. Beta HCG is the pregnancy hormone produced by the cells of the implanted embryo. As the embryo develops, beta HCG levels usually double every two days for the first several weeks. Waiting for the results of my beta was a nail-biting experience. My worry was for naught and, like some of my patients whose betas did not exactly double on schedule, I delivered a healthy baby. Consider that the precise time at which you get a blood test may not be when a growth spurt happens and, at that point, your beta has not yet doubled—but it will.

Avoiding negative self-talk

I found the first three months of pregnancy to be the most challenging and I counsel my patients to avoid negative self-talk during this time, especially if they've miscarried in the past or have been dealing with fertility issues for a long time. I suggest taking a few moments to write down your negative thoughts. These thoughts can increase your anxiety and make you depressed. Emotional stress and continuous severe depression can negatively affect pregnancy.[11] Writing your negative thoughts down can help you release them, and let go of the stress.

When you encounter bleeding

You can't help but be alarmed and fearful of a miscarriage when you see vaginal bleeding, no matter how little there is. Sometimes it does mean a miscarriage, but I've seen hundreds of women at our clinic, myself included, who have bleeding during their first trimester but end up giving birth to a healthy baby. Bleeding can be caused by:

- Progesterone suppositories. This can cause irritation in the uterine lining, resulting in bleeding, typically spotting. In clinical practice, I find up to forty percent of patients who use progesterone hormone supplements during pregnancy, or have gone through IUI or IVF, experience vaginal bleeding. Yet most of these women carry to term.

- *Subchorionic hemorrhaging* (SCH). This is a pooling of blood between the embryo and the uterine wall. It can be reabsorbed over time or resolved through vaginal bleeding (from spotting to blood clots). At one point, Barb emailed me to say she was experiencing some spotting. I told her it may be perfectly normal, but, to be safe, she should get an ultrasound. The doctor confirmed she had a subchorionic hemorrhage, but her baby was doing well.

There was not much she could do except lie low and expect to continue spotting or even have vaginal bleeding with blood clots. Several days later, she told me she'd passed a clot the size of a plum. Terrified she'd miscarried, she went for an ultrasound, which reassured her that the baby was okay and the blood clot had decreased in size. We continued with acupuncture to help her keep calm, and her uterus relaxed. She stopped bleeding and, one month later, her follow-up ultrasound showed the blood clot had disappeared.

Inadequate diet

You've had a pristine diet prior to conceiving and feel the need to eat super healthy, but you are also feeling sickly and too tired to cook. All you can get down your throat is bread, crackers, and sweets. You feel guilty and worry about harming your baby.

Don't fret. Your baby will be fine. Your body is burning extra fuel to create the superhighways of blood vessels that will feed your developing baby (or babies, if you are expecting twins). Try snacking on fresh fruits and protein (like hummus, nuts and nut butters, and cheese) every several hours to keep your blood sugar and energy level steady while providing fuel for you and your growing baby. Drink plenty of water by sipping, not guzzling. If you can't tolerate water or feel too nauseous drinking it, carbonated water (with lemon or a little juice) or ginger tea can do the trick.

Fear of flying

Flying does not have a negative impact during pregnancy for the most part.[12] In fact, there are more miscarriages related to shift work, being on your feet long periods (eight hours plus), and bending at the waist more than twenty-five times per day than there are to flying.

At one point in my fertility journey, I was pregnant with an embryo that stopped developing around six weeks (as confirmed by an ultrasound at seven weeks). Because I was awaiting an inevitable miscarriage, and we were scheduled to fly to Florida and back (three hours in each direction), I wanted to do a little science experiment and see if flying would induce a miscarriage. It didn't. I only miscarried when I took matters in my own hands twelve hours after our return and did acupuncture to induce it.

What I've learned first-hand and through the experiences of my patients is that flying is pretty safe, although I do not recommend it during the third trimester. However, trust your instincts. If you don't feel comfortable flying, don't do it, because if anything does happen, you may be tempted to blame yourself. For example, if you've never been on an airplane, it's probably not a good idea to start while you are pregnant.

Barbara's happy little ending

One last thing that's important to remember: Your doctor's job is to look for pathology and give you facts and statistics. Unfortunately, this leaves little room for hand-holding and emotional support. Instead, he may (unintentionally) scare you by comparing your developing baby to statistical norms. By the time you see a TCM practitioner, you're a mess and the practitioner must spend a lot of time trying to put you back together.

For example, one day Barb came in crying after an ultrasound during which her doctor said the baby was looking too small compared to the statistical norm and she should prepare herself for a possible miscarriage. He didn't say she would miscarry, but that was what she heard. This led her to great upset, worry, anxiety, and fear.

It's important to remember that when your doctor says these things, he or she is talking about science. Although science aims to unlock the secrets of the universe, it is not omnipotent, and neither is your doctor. Neither science nor your doctor can predict what will happen. Life is a miracle and we are each more than a set of numbers.

So when Barb came in crying after her ultrasound, I said, "I hate to break it to you, but I've met your husband. Neither of you are very tall. It's likely you will have a petite baby." Because she was focused on her doctor's words and statistics, she overlooked this simple fact. I watched her face transform as she went from panic to calm. With a sigh of relief, she told me she herself was born small—four pounds at full term. I suggested she reframe what her doctor was telling her.

After that, every time she went to her obstetrician and he said she wasn't gaining enough weight and the baby was too small, she kept her sanity and pictured a healthy little baby in her belly. And that's exactly what she got when she delivered Siera—a beautiful baby girl, weighing in at a petite but healthy five pounds and one ounce.

5

The Male Factor

Acceptance doesn't mean resignation.
It means understanding that something is what
it is and there's got to be a way through it.
MICHAEL J. FOX

Sherry and Daniel: Male factor infertility

Sherry was thirty-six when she came to see me after one failed
IVF cycle. She and her husband, Daniel, had been trying to conceive for two and a half years. In addition to having a low sperm
count, Daniel's sperm had low motility and poor morphology,
meaning they were poor swimmers and were misshapen. His
semen analysis showed he would have little or no chance of
impregnating Sherry naturally.

They opted for IVF with intracytoplasmic sperm injection
(ICSI), where semen is studied under a microscope and a
healthy sperm is injected into each mature egg. This procedure
bypasses the male factor problem, yet for them it didn't result
in pregnancy.

At a follow-up appointment, the doctor told Sherry her
eggs were shrivelled and brown—the worst he'd seen under a
microscope—and she was peri-menopausal. As if the IVF and
ICSI hadn't been enough of an ordeal, hearing that she was

prematurely menopausal felt unbearable. Even though they both had fertility challenges, it suddenly seemed to Sherry that the focus had shifted from Daniel's problem to hers. The only recommendation the doctor made was more cycles of IVF.

Together, Sherry and I acknowledged the stress, worry, and anxiety that had been building inside her, and discussed the importance of physical and emotional self-nurturing. Counselling and acupuncture helped Sherry begin to release the shock and trauma of the doctor's words.

Because it takes about 120 days for an ovulating egg to mature from a pre-antral follicle cell and sixty-four days for sperm to mature, Sherry and Daniel agreed to work with me for three months to create a healthy, nurturing, and welcoming environment in Sherry's ovaries and Daniel's gonads. This meant improving blood flow to their reproductive organs and lowering their oxidative stress by limiting their exposure to toxins, pollutants and chemicals. (Oxidative stress is like metal rusting when exposed to air. When caused by toxins, it can damage cells, including eggs and sperm.)

I devised an intensive yet relaxing treatment plan for Sherry, which included twice weekly acupuncture, changes to her diet, and some Chinese herbal medicines. Because she commuted over an hour to and from work daily, and had early morning cycle monitoring as well, she arranged to work from home several times per week, reducing her stress further.

I recommended acupuncture and Chinese herbs and supplements for Daniel to address his low sperm count and motility, as well as the malformation of his sperm. When he finally came in several months after Sherry had begun treatment, I discovered he was an avid cyclist who'd had recurrent bacterial infections over the previous eight months. These had made him violently ill for eight days with symptoms including nausea, vomiting, and acid buildup in his stomach. Being sick with fever, in addition to wearing biking shorts for prolonged periods, may have increased his scrotal temperature, thus compromising his sperm production and quality.

After several months, Sherry looked and felt better. Her bowel movements became regular, her pre-menstrual headaches stopped, and her energy increased as she slept better through the night. Daniel, who'd changed his way of eating and started cross-training instead of just cycling, was feeling better too. They also strengthened their relationship by going for walks after dinner on the days Sherry worked at home, which allowed them to connect in a way they hadn't since they were first married.

What is male factor infertility?

If a man cannot successfully impregnate his partner, his sperm will be tested for its quality and quantity, and he may be diagnosed with male factor infertility (MFI). The following problems can impede sperm's ability to fertilize an egg:

- Low sperm count (concentration of sperm). Statistically, the minimum concentration or volume required for natural conception is 20 million sperm per millilitre (mL) or per cubic centimetre (cc).[1] A man who is not producing sperm at all has *azoospermia*.
- Low motility (impaired ability to swim). To fertilize an egg, sperm must swim upstream from the cervix to the fallopian tubes, where they wait to penetrate the matured egg. Low motility will not get the sperm where they need to be to fertilize the egg.
- Poor morphology (size and shape). A normal sperm looks like a tadpole: it has a head, a mid-piece, and a tail, all of which perform specific functions. The enzymatic protein in the head penetrates the egg; the mid-piece contains

mitochondria, which fuel the cell; and the tail's whip-like action propels it upstream. Misshapen sperm may not be able to swim or to penetrate the egg.

If you are under thirty-five and not pregnant after a year of trying, or over thirty-five and not pregnant after six months of trying, you and your partner should both be tested, as it's equally likely for either of you to have fertility challenges.

Testing a man is simple. When our fertility clinic tested my husband, he ejaculated into a plastic bottle provided by the clinic in the comfort of our bathroom before work in the morning. I kept the sample at body temperature by shoving the container into my bra, between my breasts, while I drove it to the clinic. The clinic then conducted the basic tests of sperm count, motility, and morphology.

What causes male factor infertility?

The following causes of MFI are related to genetic and anatomical abnormalities, or in some cases disease, and are therefore beyond the individual's control:

- Varicoceles, or varicose veins in the scrotum, can affect sperm production. The most common cause of MFI, varicoceles occurs in fifteen percent of the normal male population (without MFI) and about forty percent of men presenting with fertility challenges.[2] Forty-two percent of men over sixty have varicoceles.[3] In my practice, I have seen some men get women pregnant naturally in spite of having it.
- Orchitis, swelling and inflammation of the testicles, can impede sperm production. Orchitis can result from having mumps, birth defects of the urinary tract, sexually transmitted infections (STI), or bacterial infections from medical instruments.

- Cystic fibrosis. Simply being a carrier of CF can cause the vas deferens, a part of the male reproductive organ, to be missing.
- Klinefelter syndrome, where a man is born with an extra X chromosome (XXY instead of XY), causing sterility.
- Undescended testicles, where the testicles do not drop down from the abdomen during fetal development, can be surgically repaired at birth but can still lead to sterility.
- Vasectomy reversal, which can cause production of sperm antibodies.
- Chemotherapy or radiation. Chemo targets and quickly kills dividing cells such as sperm and can damage immature cells in the testes. Radiation, if carried out near the scrotum, will kill sperm cells as well as cancer cells.
- Kidney disease, which often leads to cysts in the seminal vesicle, can impact semen parameters and can rarely lead to *azoospermia* (no sperm in semen).[4]
- Retrograde ejaculation, where semen backs up into the bladder, can be a congenital issue. Alternatively, it can occur post-surgically or be caused by medications.
- Genetic problems, like *chromosomal translocation,* which is thoroughly explained in Chapter 7.
- Any acute or chronic inflammatory disease, particularly if it leads to an episode of high fever.

In addition, the following factors in MFI are lifestyle issues and very much within the individual's control:

- Alcohol consumption. This may decrease sperm count and quality, and cause DNA fragmentation (see next page).[5]
- Drug use (including prescription, some over-the-counter, and street drugs). Some drugs, such as cannabis, can reduce sperm motility and decrease its ability to penetrate eggs.[6]

- Cigarette smoking.[7] Tobacco can cause oxidative stress, which can damage genetic material.
- Weight. A high body-mass index (BMI), which is a weight-to-height ratio, can lower semen volume, as well as sperm concentration, sperm count, and sperm motility, though there appears to be no effect on morphology (shape).[8]
- Diabetes. This can alter endocrine function, increase oxidative stress, impede blood flow to the testicles, and therefore damage sperm.[9] While some diabetes is type 1, and therefore beyond the individual's control, more commonly these days it is the result of poor diet and therefore a lifestyle factor.
- Increased scrotal temperature. This can result from being sick with a fever, which may be beyond one's control, although fever-reducing medications can help. But using a laptop for prolonged periods with nothing to absorb the heat;[10] sitting in saunas, steam baths, or hot tubs for extended periods;[11] or wearing tight briefs or cycling tights[12] can also raise scrotal temperature and affect sperm production.
- Exposure to toxins. Chemicals such as Bisphenol-A, which can leach from hard plastics, such as water bottles, into foods, can decrease sperm count, concentration, and motility.[13]

Other male factors in infertility

Other male infertility factors, including DNA fragmentation and immune factors, require additional testing. *DNA fragmentation* refers to breaks in the sperm's genetic blueprint; while the sperm may be able to fertilize an egg, it may impact the health of an ongoing pregnancy, such as by increasing risk of miscarriage. DNA fragmentation of greater than twenty-five percent renders sperm *sub-fertile*.[14]

Urologist Dr. Paul Turek explains DNA fragmentation this way: "Think of chromosomal imbalances as men with two left feet and fragmented sperm DNA as men with shoes on the wrong feet. Either way, the dance (with the egg for fertilization) just isn't as smooth as it should be and it just stops in its tracks."[15]

MFI can also be immunological. Sometimes a man produces sperm antibodies that prevent his sperm from penetrating an egg. Normally, sperm is isolated and produced within the testes away from the rest of a man's body without contact. But if there is a break in the barrier, as can happen after trauma to the gonads (like being kicked hard) or surgeries such as vasectomy reversal (reconnection of male reproductive tract after steriliza- tion), the body produces antibodies to sperm, which fight them off and kill them as if they were foreign invaders.

MFI can also be *idiopathic*, which means it appears to hap- pen spontaneously, without an identifiable cause. For example, hormonal issues due to a problem in the hypothalamic-pituitary- gonadal axis can cause a breakdown anywhere from the brain to the gonads (such as low testosterone), which can impede sperm production. However, while this can be idiopathic, it can also be related to lifestyle issues, and therefore is some- times possible to treat.

How common is male factor infertility?

Male factor infertility accounts for approximately forty percent of fertility issues, female infertility accounts for another thirty to forty percent, and twenty percent can result from the com- bined fertility issues of both partners. The balance is unexplained infertility (see Chapter 1).[16]

Although men are as likely to have fertility issues as women, male patients account for less than five percent of the fertility treatments in my Chinese medical practice. Even when there is a male factor issue, it's usually the female partner who seeks help while the male stays at home. I reached out to thirty TCM practitioners around North America and found they all had similar statistics. One practitioner in San Francisco said she sees virtually no men for fertility issues.

I can see two reasons for this. First, we know how difficult it can be for women to be open about their fertility challenges, but it's even more difficult for men because of the assumption that a "real" man is virile and can father a child any time after puberty. One of my female patients said, "It's like I'm questioning his manhood by suggesting that our problem conceiving is just as likely to originate with him." Many patients tell me that talking about their man's possible role in fertility challenges shakes his self-esteem and he sometimes begins avoiding intimacy altogether.

Second, on some level, science and technology absolve men of the need to take any responsibility for fertility. So even when a couple's problem originates with the male, it's typically the woman who receives treatment.

Take the lead

It can be very frustrating for women to constantly assume the onus of keeping things going, because if they don't, nothing will happen. In my case, if I hadn't kept the ball in the air, my husband would have let it fall and walked away. He figured we had a good life, we could travel and do things we wanted, anywhere, anytime, so why mess with it. It's not that he didn't want children. He did, and he was good with kids. It was just difficult for him to watch me go through all the drugs, procedures, and emotional and physical suffering in order to conceive. Consequently, it seemed as though I was always about five steps ahead of him, like many of the couples I see who are thinking about building a family.

That meant I, like other women, was willing to subject myself to more lifestyle changes, discomfort, and even indignities to have a child than my husband, who was resistant and complained every step of the way. In the end, he supported my decision, and let me

decide how long we would continue down this pathway toward creating a family. It took six to eight months for me to digest the fact
that my fallopian tubes were blocked and the only way we were
going to get pregnant was if I surrendered to IVF. But now we're both
grateful I did because Zoe would not be here today otherwise.

It's funny how women can totally alter their lifestyle habits,
while many of their partners barely change anything. For some, it's
one of the most frustrating things a woman has to deal with. It's like
walking on eggshells: you're seething inside because you are doing
all you can while (without over-generalizing) he's still drinking beer
and eating pizza. You don't want to cause a rift in your relationship
and you don't want to nag, but whatever you say, even with good
intentions, your partner likely will not want to hear it. Maybe this
is why men don't have uteruses!

IUI/IVF: The quick fixes

With any of the aforementioned sperm issues, assisted reproductive technology (ART) can provide quick solutions (at least
from the male perspective). This goes back to the second reason
most men do not come to see me for fertility issues. As long as
they can ejaculate into a cup, their problem is solved.

Even if they can't produce on demand, if there is little sperm
in the ejaculate, or if the sperm is damaged, the doctor can grab
some healthy sperm using a small needle inserted into either
the testicles (testicular sperm aspiration, or TESA) or the vas
deferens (percutaneous epididymal sperm aspiration, or PESA).
If there is no sperm production at all, the doctor can perform
a surgery called testicular sperm extraction (TESE) to extract
small amounts of tissue from the testes to look for sperm.

Obtaining sperm any of these ways allows a couple to bypass
sex completely. After observing the sperm under a microscope,
the embryologist chooses good-looking, fast, straight-swimming

sperm and injects a single sperm directly into each matured egg during IVF with ICSI.

In my opinion, this technology is both a blessing and a curse. It is extraordinary that modern science has come so far as to enable men with physical factors like cystic fibrosis, spinal cord injury, or post-chemotherapy fertility issues to pass their genes on to their offspring. However, I also believe fertility clinics can be quick to use technology instead of focusing on educating men whose lifestyle choices have caused or contributed to their MFI about the natural steps they can take to enhance the quality and quantity of their sperm production or address sexual dysfunction.

It seems to me that fertility clinics avoid treating these men's underlying problems because their job is to help them get a baby in their partner's belly, not to worry about the quality and health of the couple's sex life. I have also heard from female patients that they felt as if fertility doctors were more sensitive to male egos, wanting men to feel good about themselves despite their fertility challenges. My patients reported that fertility doctors said more encouraging things to men, minimizing their problems conceiving a child and reassuring them about the simplicity of conceiving a child using IUI or IVF. Not only does this approach allow men to avoid addressing their own, manageable issues; they also require their female partners to undergo the stress of IUI or IVF.

Changing the sperm's environment

I view sperm production the same way I see egg production: grown in the right environment, sperm parameters can change. Our external and internal environments, and the way we react to them, can have a huge impact on our bodies. What we eat, how we move, and the way we think can all affect the physical environment in which sperm are produced.

One of my patients and her partner both had fertility testing done and were shocked to learn that while his sperm count and motility were normal, eighty-nine percent of his sperm were abnormally shaped, making it impossible for them to penetrate an egg. He typically smoked one or two personal-sized joints per day for ten years to help him unwind and relax. I suggested to Cindy that he quit smoking pot to see what happened.

A month later he had his sperm retested. Its parameters were completely normal and Cindy became pregnant naturally a few months later. Changing something that's been an important part of a person's lifestyle for a decade is never simple, yet this was a case where one difficult change by the male made a huge difference, and saved his partner from going through the stress, trauma, and cost of fertility treatments that usually focus on the woman.

As with women, I believe it's important for men to eat well, beginning with whole, organic, unprocessed foods. The expression "You are what you eat" means that what you eat can have an impact on every cell in your body—including your sperm.

For one study, a group of young men between eighteen and twenty-two were divided into two groups over a year. The men who ate more fish, chicken, fruit, vegetables, legumes, and whole grains had faster-swimming sperm compared with those who ate a lot of red and processed meat, refined grains, pizza, snacks, high-energy drinks, and sweets.[17] I believe better nutrients provide more fuel and, hence, faster sperm. The young men who ate the more processed diet showed no negative effects on their semen quality, but I'm guessing that, if they were to continue eating the same way and tracking their sperm parameters for ten or twenty years, more of those in the unhealthy food group would be struggling with MFI than in the healthy food group.

Along similar lines, studies have shown that following a Mediterranean diet—which focuses on fruits, vegetables, whole grains, legumes, olive oil, and lean proteins such as fish and poultry, as well as including regular servings of red wine (consumed in moderation)—increases sperm potential.[18]

Certain foods also contain estrogens, which can negatively affect sperm parameters. For example, dairy has been known to contain large amounts of estrogens, which is associated with poor semen quality, specifically morphology.[19] So limit dairy, but when you do eat and drink it, find a non-hormonally treated source. Likewise, soy estrogen is not so good for males (or females). However, eat lots of fruits and vegetables, as the antioxidants protect the cells against damage.

Here is a list of dos and don'ts to protect sperm health:

- Reduce coffee intake. The Department of Urology at Cornell Medical College recommends one to two cups per day. There is no conclusive evidence that coffee damages sperm, but looking at it from a TCM perspective, we say to do things in moderation. Coffee lovers can decrease their intake and buy organic, pesticide-free coffee. If they can cut it to half a cup per day or just have it as a treat occasionally, so much the better.
- Do not smoke. Smoking causes oxidative damage to cells.[20]
- Do not drink more than two ounces of alcohol per week. In a study, men who had six ounces of hard liquor (forty to fifty percent alcohol) five days per week for a year had lowered testosterone and progesterone levels, and increased levels of FSH, estrogen, and LH, which lowered sperm parameters in volume, count, motility, and morphology.[21]
- Exercise moderately to release stress. As with women, accumulated stress may impede energy flow to reproductive organs. Moderate exercise allows energy and blood to flow

through the body, whereas vigorous exercise can over-consume energy that could go toward sperm production.

- Watch your weight. In a study, overweight men (BMI 25–29.9 kg/m2) had decreased semen volume; obese men (BMI 30–40 kg/m2) had not only decreased semen volume but also fewer motile sperm (good swimmers)[22] and an increased number of chromosomal abnormalities.[23]

- Manage stress. In a study that compared men who experienced two or more stressful life events (like a death in the family) within a year with men who had experienced no stressful events in the same time period, the former had a lower percentage of motile sperm and morphologically normal sperm, even though they had a similar sperm concentration. Job strain was not associated with semen parameters, although it was found that employed men had higher sperm concentration overall with more motile sperm and more morphologically normal sperm than unemployed men.[24]

- Minimize exposure to toxins like PCBs in farmed fatty fish, Bisphenol-A in plastics and canned foods, pesticides, lead, pollutants, and ozone. They cause oxidative stress and DNA damage to sperm.[25] A study showed that occupational exposure to toxic solvents, heavy metals, heat, vibrations, and non-ionizing radiation increased risk factors that affected sperm parameters. This would apply to labourers, painters, farmers, welders, plumbers, and technicians.[26]

- Do not overheat testicles. Nature positioned the scrotum away from the body because sperm are produced in a slightly cooler environment than core body temperature. Therefore:

  > In general, men should stay away from saunas, steam baths, or hot tubs for long periods of time. A study showed that having a sauna set between 80 and 90 degrees Celsius twice weekly for fifteen minutes each time for

three months affected sperm production, which is also the length of time it takes for a sperm to mature.[27] If a sauna or steam bath helps with relaxation, there's no problem with enjoying it occasionally. But men with fertility challenges should make it snappy, not do it too often, and take a cool shower afterwards.

> Men with fertility concerns should keep laptops off their laps and cell phones away from the groin since they can increase the temperature in the area by 2.75 degrees Celsius (5 degrees Fahrenheit) over core body temperature (even one degree over core body temperature can have a negative impact on sperm production).[28]

> Men should store cell phones away from front pant pockets since studies have found that exposure for more than four hours per day can damage sperm DNA.[29]

• Limit time wearing biking tights or shorts. The constriction decreases scrotal blood flow. A study showed men who biked more than five hours per week had more than four percent less motile sperm (good swimmers) than those who did not (12.1 percent vs. 16.4 percent).[30]

• Brush and floss teeth. Bacteria from gum disease and bad oral hygiene can enter the blood stream, infecting semen and causing subfertility in men.[31]

• If possible, avoid the following prescription medications.[32] Consult your doctor to discuss alternative drugs that may have less impact on fertility. Otherwise, use your doctor's guidance to find the minimum dose you can take. Do not go off medication without consulting your doctor first.

> Tricyclic antidepressants. Although rarely used to treat depression anymore, they are commonly prescribed at low doses to control chronic pain.

> Steroids, which are sometimes used to reduce inflammation that causes pain or asthma. In some cases, steroids

can be injected directly into local pain sites, reducing risk to fertility.

> Calcium channel blockers, which increase blood and oxygen to the heart.
> Allopurinol, which decreases uric acid buildup and is used to treat and prevent kidney stones and gout.
> Cimetidine, which decreases stomach acid and helps with stomach and duodenal ulcers and pain.
> Alpha blockers, which open and relax blood vessels to treat high blood pressure.
> Sulfasalazine, which decreases intestinal inflammation in ulcerative colitis.
> Nitrofurantoin, an antibiotic used to treat UTI.
> Valproic acid, an anti-seizure medication also used to treat bipolar disorder and migraines.
> Lithium, used to prevent manic episodes associated with bipolar disorder.
> Spironolactone or "water pills," used to treat high blood pressure and edema.
> Colchicine, used in the treatment of gout.
> Antipsychotics, which block receptors in the brain to treat mania and schizophrenia,
> Finasteride (Propecia, Proscar), which helps to shrink an enlarged prostate.
> Testosterone supplements, which are used to treat deficiencies of male hormones associated with male sexual characteristics.

Epigenetics in MFI

As mentioned earlier, when a female partner doesn't get pregnant, the onus still seems to fall on her, because she is deemed a "poor responder" or "her eggs are getting older" or she has an autoimmune issue that is causing her body to reject the sperm or embryo.

But it takes two to tango. MFI alone contributes to almost half of fertility issues, and sperm factors like DNA fragmentation contribute to up to thirty percent of recurrent miscarriages. Also, although there's a belief that men remain virile virtually without limit, advancing age for a fellow can decrease success rates of IVF and IUI while increasing rates of preterm births, autism, childhood leukemia, schizophrenia, bipolar disorder, and cleft lip.[33] Just as eggs can get older and need more care, so can sperm. The good news is that sperm problems, like egg problems, don't have to be permanent. As the science of epigenetics tells us, any cell, including eggs and sperm, can grow to its full potential given the right environment. So the onus should not be just on the woman to take charge of her health. A man can too.

From what we know, DNA fragmentation tests are current to a specific time and sample. Because men's bodies generate about 1200 new sperm per second,[34] DNA fragmentation levels can change from week to week, and can be affected by a man's emotional environment as well as physical exposure to heat, drugs, and toxicity. Such environmental exposures over time and with advancing age can lead to improper sperm formation and mutate the genes impacting the offspring's health and development physically and behaviorally for the next two generations (or more, depending on the toxic exposures or nutritional deficiencies).[35] For example:

- Men who take opiates (morphine-like drugs, usually used as painkillers but sometimes recreationally) before conception can cause developmental and behavioural impairments in their offspring. In some cases, these problems can be transmitted through the male line to the second and third generations (not only the son but the grandson and even the great-grandson).[36]

- If the father's nutritional environment is poor, as in the case of famine, his offspring's cells may thrive efficiently in a scarcity environment but when born and exposed to normal amounts of food, he may develop metabolic syndrome, in which the body stores food as fat in preparation for the next famine. This increases risk of obesity, high blood pressure, heart disease, and stroke in the offspring.[37]

Supplements and sperm

Our overall food supply isn't what it used to be. Think about this: when you pick a fruit ripe off a tree, it is juicy and sweet. But if you pick the same fruit before its prime, and then truck-ripen it as it journeys to wherever it's being shipped, you can taste the difference. The fruit is less flavourful because it is less developed. This is one reason I believe in supplementation.

Try finding a male supplement that contains antioxidants and nutrients good for sperm formation. It should include the following:[38]

- Vitamin C, 1000 mg/day (500 mg twice a day), has been shown to prevent DNA damage, when combined with Vitamin E, 1000 IU (500 IU twice per day).[39]
- L-Carnitine and Acetyl-L-Carnitine, 145 mg per day and 64 mg per day, respectively, prevent sperm damage, improve sperm quality, and help sperm swim faster.[40]
- Selenium, 80–200 mcg per day, has been shown to protect against sperm damage and support sperm function.[41]
- Zinc sulfate, 10 mg per day, supports sperm formation and morphology, and protects again oxidative stress.[42]
- CoQ10, 200 mg per day, provides fuel for cells and has been shown to support sperm formation.[43]
- Folic acid, 200 mcg per day of methylated folate, has been shown to boost sperm count.[44]

- Vitamin B12 (cyanocobalamin), 1 mcg daily, has been shown to maintain blood health.[45]
- Lycopene, 6 mg per day, has been shown to prevent DNA damage (fragmentation).[46]

Sherry and Daniel and baby makes three

After three months of working with me, Sherry and Daniel attempted another IVF cycle. This time, when the doctor retrieved Sherry's eggs, he was amazed to see that they looked normal and asked her what she had been doing to bring about such a dramatic change. At the same time, Daniel's sample showed that his sperm count had increased from 1 to 10 million. Although this is still considered less than normal, it was ten times more than it had been at his last test.

The IVF cycle did not result in a pregnancy, but Sherry and Daniel felt less devastated. In fact, they felt more in control in their health, knowing their lifestyle changes and taking charge of their health had been a step in the right direction. They tried a third cycle of IVF unsuccessfully before taking a break from the physical, psychological, and financial stress of going to the fertility clinic.

But we continued treatments as they made their lifestyle changes permanent, and they continued living their lives. A year later, Sherry spontaneously conceived and gave birth to her miracle girl, Elisa.

Gail and Justin: Delayed ejaculation

Gail and Justin were another couple I worked with, but their issues were quite different. At thirty-eight, Gail had perfect periods, with a twenty-eight-day cycle that never wavered. This made it easy to time intercourse, as ovulation occurs fourteen days before menstruation and, technically, a woman's most fertile days are four to five days prior to and at ovulation.

Gail made sure they were having sex from days nine to fifteen to cover their bases. But her husband had delayed ejaculation (DE), and his greatest difficulty was ejaculating through partner sex. They'd been trying unsuccessfully to conceive for almost a year when they went to a fertility clinic.

Justin had no trouble ejaculating manually, so the clinic suggested they try home insemination, injecting semen into Gail's vagina with a syringe. After trying this method unsuccessfully for six months, they opted for IVF. These were all ways for Justin to bypass his issues with delayed ejaculation, meaning Gail had to undergo treatment at the fertility clinic herself.

What is delayed ejaculation?

DE occurs when a man has a normal erection but is unable to ejaculate through sexual intercourse, as was the case for Justin. This can lead to a technical challenge because the sperm do not go through the vagina to meet the egg. It can be mild, where men are only able to ejaculate after thirty to forty minutes of intercourse and with great effort. In a more severe form, a man can only ejaculate by himself and not even in the presence of his sexual partner. In the most severe cases, a man has never been able to ejaculate (*anejaculatory*). DE impairs fertility because the sperm does not go into the vagina. However, DE can also severely affect a couple's sexual enjoyment because male orgasm is not reached in a timely way, or at all.[47]

What causes DE?

Common psychological causes of DE as documented by the Mayo Clinic[48] and US National Library of Medicine[49] include:

- Conditioning through excessive masturbation.
- Traumatic events (could be emotional, like having been cheated on by a partner).

- Depression, anxiety, or other mental health conditions.
- Relationship issues due to stress, lack of attraction for partner, or poor communication.
- Anxiety about performance.
- Poor body image.
- Cultural or religious taboos regarding sex.
- Differences between sex with a partner and sexual fantasies.
- Emotional factors, such as anger toward the partner.

Physical causes may include:

- Blockage of the ducts that semen passes through.
- Use of certain drugs, such as some antidepressants, antipsychotics, anti-seizure drugs, or drugs for high blood pressure.
- Use of alcohol, particularly to excess (alcohol abuse or alcoholism).
- Nervous system diseases, such as stroke or nerve damage to the spinal cord or back.
- Testosterone deficiency.
- Nerve damage during surgery to the pelvis.
- Certain birth defects affecting the male reproductive system.
- Injury to the pelvic nerves that control orgasm.
- Certain infections, such as urinary tract infections.
- Prostate surgery, such as *transurethral resection of the prostate* (TURP) or prostate removal.
- Neurological diseases, such as diabetic neuropathy, stroke, or nerve damage to the spinal cord.
- Hormone-related conditions, such as *hypothyroidism* (low thyroid hormone) or *hypogonadism* (low testosterone).
- *Retrograde ejaculation*, a condition in which the semen goes backward into the bladder rather than out of the penis.

Maintaining intimacy despite delayed ejaculation or erectile dysfunction

It can be challenging to maintain intimacy in your relationship while dealing with any fertility challenges. Here are a few things that have helped my patients, as well as my husband and me, through this journey. The good news is, in a loving and lasting relationship, intimacy does not always mean sexual intercourse:

- Holding hands while walking together or watching television.
- Saying "I love you" every day.
- Hugging several times a day. I say a good squeeze for at least twenty seconds stimulates release of oxytocin, the love hormone. But according to the late Virginia Satir, an American psychologist and family therapist, "we need four hugs a day for survival, eight a day for maintenance and 12 a day for growth."[50]
- Kissing, from long, passionate, hot kisses to little kisses on the lips and face, helps to keep you close. (My husband and I made a rule in our household to kiss ten times a day. We also have a rule to never go to bed mad at each other. Anger stored over time creates distance rather than intimacy.)
- Rae Dolman, a sexologist in Toronto, recommends making time for each other by going out on dates or having in-house dates like watching a movie or making a nice dinner.
- Dolman also advocates communicating consciously, which means taking the blame out of everything. Instead of saying, "You do this and that," start by saying, "When you do this (fact), I feel this way." This brings responsibility to your communication without blame while respecting and showing empathy for your partner.

What is erectile dysfunction?

Erectile dysfunction (ED), also known as impotence, is the consistent inability to achieve or maintain an erection for sexual activity over a three-month period. More than 150 million men worldwide live with ED, and it's been predicted that it will affect about 250 million men by 2025.[51] In the United States, more than eighteen percent of men (18 million) over twenty years old experience long-term ED. ED increases with age, but it correlates more to age-related health issues like high blood pressure, diabetes, and heart disease than to age itself.[52] More than half of American men with ED have diabetes.[53]

ED in itself is not considered an infertility problem because a man experiencing ED can have normal sperm count, motility, and morphology. However, difficulty in achieving and sustaining enough of an erection for penetration and ejaculation can pose a physical challenge for couples trying to conceive. ED can also stress the hypothalamic-pituitary-gonadal axis, impeding the cascade of hormones involved in producing sperm. That means that a man's anxiety about being unable to achieve and sustain an erection can affect his brain's ability to trigger the appropriate hormonal response and blood flow required for sperm production. In this case, there is a direct correlation between ED and male infertility.[54]

Many couples having these issues think they are alone, but men at any age can experience ED occasionally. If it happens less than twenty percent of the time, there's likely no need to seek professional help. As men age, they experience ED more, because the blood vessels that supply the penis grow narrower and the blood flow required to achieve full erection diminishes. In younger men, stress, anxiety, and depression can interfere with blood flow, because if a man is in fight-or-flight mode, his energy and blood are redirected to his head, heart, and limbs rather than his penis.

What causes ED?

Rae Dolman tells me she sees men with ED who have an otherwise clean bill of health more than fifty percent of the time. Men with ED and DE comprise a third of her patient population, while the other third are female, and the last third are couples. ED can arise from any of the following physical or emotional factors:

- Alcohol consumption. Alcohol is a depressant, and in excess it can impair sexual function.
- Cigarette smoking. This increases risk of high blood pressure and atherosclerosis, which affects blood vessels.
- Depression, anger, anxiety, and stress. As noted above, these trigger a stress response, which diverts blood away from the reproductive organs.
- Prescription drug use. Drugs for blood pressure and depression can cause ED, but do not attempt to stop taking medications without consulting your doctor first.
- Street drug use. Amphetamines, cocaine, and marijuana can all contribute to ED.
- Obesity or being overweight. Excess weight is often correlated with reduced male sex hormones and increases the risk of hypertension and atherosclerosis, which can impede blood flow to the penis.
- Low libido. The above factors can also lead to low libido, and if you are not in the mood, it dampens the ability to "get it up." Another cause for diminished sex drive is low testosterone. In Chinese medicine, low libido can come from a deficiency of kidney Jing essence, the energy that rules the reproductive hormones. This depletion may come from overworking physically or emotionally, or from excessive sexual activity (depleting essence through sperm).
- Diabetes, hypertension, atherosclerosis, and cardiovascular disease. All these conditions can impede blood flow, as can

cardiovascular risk factors such as high total cholesterol levels and low high-density lipoprotein cholesterol levels.

- Spinal cord injuries. These can cause ED, depending on the nature of the injury.
- Multiple sclerosis. MS is a neurological dysfunction that can impact proper sexual function. As well, psychological factors or generalized MS symptoms, such as fatigue, muscular weakness, and urination problems, can cause ED. Side effects of medications for MS can also contribute.[55]
- Surgery to treat prostate or bladder problems. This can affect the nerves and blood vessels that control erection.

Gail and Justin and twins make four

I supported Gail with weekly acupuncture and she took prescribed herbal medicines to help enhance the quality of her eggs. She became pregnant with her first IVF but miscarried. After her second IVF, she conceived again and miraculously gave birth to healthy identical twins, Aiden and Tom.

Gail and her husband didn't view his DE as a problem in their relationship. They believed their relationship was solid and that they still had good sex—just without orgasm through partner sex. They found the best way to show their love for each other was to practice intimacy without sex.

6

Making the Workplace Work for Fertility

Vulnerability is not weakness, it's emotional risk,
exposure, and the most accurate measure of courage.
BRENE BROWN

Samantha: Polycystic ovarian syndrome (PCOS)

Samantha was thirty-two when she came to see me. She and
her husband, Devan, had immigrated to Canada after marry-
ing in India three and a half years ago. She landed a demanding
job as a middle manager at a large corporation and gave it her
all, working long hours, often going in early and staying late.
Striving for the next promotion and raise gave her a sense of
purpose and satisfaction.

After a year and a half of marriage, Samantha, then thirty,
and Devan decided to start a family. It was challenging because
her periods became irregular after leaving India. They went to
a fertility clinic, where Samantha was told she was not ovulating
and was diagnosed with polycystic ovarian syndrome (PCOS).

The fertility doctor gave her progesterone to bring on her
period. He also prescribed Metformin, a diabetic drug to
control blood sugar levels, which is often associated with PCOS.

He then put her on Clomid, a hormone drug, to help with ovulation. She tried the Clomid for three menstrual cycles in which she had daily early morning monitoring with blood work and ultrasounds, but she did not get pregnant and became more stressed than ever.

About Metformin

More often than not, women with PCOS who are working with a fertility clinic when they show up at my door are taking Metformin whether they are insulin-resistant or not. It reduces blood sugars and male sex hormones but can have long-term negative consequences. Dr. Yaakov Bentoff, a reproductive endrocrinologist (RE) at TCART Fertility Partners in Toronto, who, unlike other REs, generally does not prescribe Metformin, explained the potentially serious implications:

"Metformin inhibits the ability of the cell to produce energy. This is the same action as but less potent than cyanide (causing cell death). Less energy means less energy to produce androgens (male hormones). The cell has to compensate for a lack of ability to produce energy in the same level of efficiency as before. So for long-term use there is a compensation mechanism causing long-term effects. When humans are given Metformin in pregnancy, it's like starvation, since the cell becomes deficient in energy. We know from very old studies that starving women while pregnant will have kids who grow up becoming obese and have all the signs of metabolic syndrome, insulin resistance, hypertension, and diabetes as adults."

As noted in Chapter 5, starving a fetus causes genetic changes resulting from environmental influences that make energy-producing mechanisms highly efficient; with very small amounts of sugar left in the blood stream, they can produce a lot of energy. But when these babies are born into the real world, where energy and nutrients are abundant, they develop *metabolic syndrome*, which can lead to diabetes and from there to hypertension and cardiovascular disease.

Metformin creates an environment like that of starvation; there is less energy, so cells become more efficient in energy production. When babies are born and away from Metformin, they develop insulin resistance, diabetes, and metabolic syndrome. At Dr. Bentoff's clinic as well as ours, we recommend lifestyle and dietary changes, which is enough to produce longstanding positive results in many cases.

What is PCOS?

PCOS is a complex condition affecting the endocrine system (the hormone-producing glands). It's diagnosed when you have two of the three following symptoms:[1]

- Excessive male steroid hormones in the body, characterized by acne, excessive body hair, or thinning hair.
- Ovulatory dysfunction, where the egg doesn't mature or release properly from the ovaries, leading to irregular or no menstruation.
- Polycystic ovaries, as seen by ultrasound.

PCOS affects six to ten percent of women of reproductive age[2] and is often associated with insulin resistance, a condition in which the body's cells do not recognize insulin, requiring the body to work harder to produce it. PCOS is also associated with glucose intolerance (high amounts of sugar in the body) and obesity. Samantha, being South Asian, was ethnically predisposed to this condition.[3] In addition, Samantha ate a vegetarian diet, heavy in white flour and white rice. Refined carbohydrates like these convert to sugar in the body, raising blood glucose levels quickly.

Normally, insulin, which is produced in the pancreas, helps store or convert sugar from the blood stream into usable energy, including energy to produce appropriate hormones and develop eggs. If the body is insulin resistant, it lacks the capacity to convert sugar to energy and instead turns it to fat, increasing the risk of hormonal dysfunction, as in PCOS, and resulting in higher male hormone levels and a reduced ability to ovulate.

Worried about work

In addition to being anxious and fearful about being unable to ovulate and conceive on her own, attending the fertility clinic almost daily for early morning cycle monitoring was affecting Samantha's work. Instead of getting to work early as usual, she arrived late every day. She'd compensate by working late, but this wasn't enough for her boss, who only saw her late arrival, not her late departure. To him, she seemed uncommitted to her job, and in this cut-throat, male-dominated company, she felt she could not tell him she was trying to have a baby. She feared not only losing out on the next raise or promotion but losing her job because pregnancy and motherhood were considered liabilities.

Instead, she told her manager she had a medical issue. As she suspected, she did not get the support she needed. She'd prided herself on her impeccable work ethic, but when her manager gave her a year-end performance review that paled in comparison with past reviews, she was beside herself. Frustrated, hurt, and angry at how little her dedication and hard work were appreciated, she lost her drive and focus, dreaded going into work each day, and resented having to work late.

I see this scenario daily. We know the stress of trying to conceive is comparable to facing a life-threatening illness, and because of the stigma surrounding it, most people keep their fertility challenges private. By the time Samantha came to see me, she was overwhelmed, depressed, and emotionally and physically hanging by a thread. She had not had a period in five months. She was socially isolated because she spent so much time at work, she had difficulty sleeping, and she had gained weight. To make matters worse, she started to lose the hair on the top of her head and developed debilitating headaches, high blood pressure, backaches, and neck and shoulder tension. She also starting having frequent colds and had difficulty concentrating.

Based on her symptoms alone, it was obvious her stress levels were affecting all parts of her body, mind, and spirit. Her fertility challenges made sense to me because she was out of balance in many areas of her life and had not been supporting a nurturing internal environment.

When I asked Samantha when she'd last felt happy, she realized she hadn't been happy since leaving India four years earlier. Her life in Canada had been all work and no play. She hadn't created a balanced lifestyle, she was working in a negative environment, and she was worried about her job security.

We need life to create life

In Chapter 3, we talked about depression evolving out of grief and unresolved emotional trauma. When our energy is drained by the heaviness of life, our survival instinct diverts our energy to where it is necessary for survival and steers it away from our reproductive organs.

When I asked Samantha about her weight, she told me she'd gained thirty pounds (over thirteen kilograms) since moving to Canada—a lot for anyone, never mind someone who's only five feet tall. Since leaving India, her lifestyle had become sedentary, sitting at her desk for hours at a time.

By the time she began going to the fertility clinic, she was finding no time to socialize, exercise, or eat properly. She'd adopted the North American habit of eating fast foods on the run. Every morning she bought a cup of coffee and a muffin, which she ate at her desk. She bought a vegetarian sandwich for lunch. At the end of her long day, she'd make a traditional Indian dinner with roti and white rice, vegetables, and lentils or chickpeas. The overload of carbohydrates impacted her sugar tolerance. Her unhealthy eating, lifestyle, and emotional stress resulted in ovulatory issues and lack of periods. To me, there is no stronger way for your body to say, "No, not now" than through an absence of menstruation.

I explained to her that by changing her lifestyle and eating habits, losing weight, and minimizing her response to emotional and physical stress, she could restore her fertility naturally. But to do so, she would need to invest time and effort in a more balanced and healthy lifestyle.

It takes a village

There is an expression that it takes a village to raise a child. I say it takes a village to make a child. If you are having fertility challenges, you need to cultivate this village as much as you need to cultivate the soil in which to plant the seed that will become a baby.

I had to devise a life-altering plan of action for Samantha that was both attainable and empowering. It encompassed creating support at home, work, and in the community, and using different forms of Chinese medicine to address her specific health issues.

At home, if you are overwhelmed, you need to ask your partner to help share in the cooking, cleaning, grocery shopping, and running errands.

Among friends and family, you need to find one person you can trust. They may not fully understand your fertility challenges, so you need to help them by telling them what you do and don't want them to say.

You also need to find professional support, such as by seeing a fertility counsellor or other therapist, trying hypnosis with someone who specializes in fertility issues, or attending a fertility support group.

Finding support at work can be tricky. Unfortunately, Samantha's work environment was toxic, and her body was chronically in survival mode. Something had to change. In her case, I recommended some time off. I told her to seek the support of her family doctor, who could assess her mental and physical health. Seeing that the challenges of trying to conceive were leading to depression, headaches, high blood pressure, difficulty concentrating, and lack of focus, her doctor wrote a letter recommending Samantha take a three-month stress leave.

I will discuss this more later in the chapter because there are different ways to navigate working while trying to conceive. In some work environments, like Samantha's, that means taking time off; other workplaces are more conducive to baby-making.

Forms of Chinese medicine

Your TCM doctor and herbalist will prescribe formulas made of dried raw herbs. These formulas are put together much like recipes, as each ingredient has different properties and therapeutic actions. These can be wide and varied, as the herbal pharmacopeia contains thousands of different herbs. They are combined into individual prescriptions that you take home, rinse, soak in water, boil, and cook for several hours. You strain and drink the reserves, divided into two servings daily. This is considered the most concentrated way of extracting the medicinal properties from the herbs.

Alternatively, you can take prepared decoctions, which are prescribed and cooked for you at a facility, and then mailed to you or picked up by you. Or you can buy granules—herbs that have been commercially cooked and concentrated, which you then reconstitute with hot water. Finally, you can buy powdered herbs, which have been cooked, dried, and powdered, and then pressed into tablets or boluses to be taken with warm water.

TCM practitioners have different opinions about the most effective forms of delivery. Freshly decocted herbs are inarguably more potent, but in my experience, the lengthy and smelly cooking process leads to lower compliance. Most individuals come to me already stressed out, so adding an expectation can send them over the edge. If taking herbs another way increases compliance, it may be more effective in the long run.

After four months of working together weekly, Samantha felt better. Her life changed. She walked daily, did yoga twice weekly, took three months off work, and changed her eating habits without dieting. She stopped eating refined sugars and instead ate fruit when she wanted something sweet. She also went to a monthly fertility support group led by a fertility counsellor, where she connected with women like her who had kept their fertility issues private.

Diet and lifestyle changes to heal PCOS

Healthy lifestyle and dietary habits are crucial for helping PCOS. In Chapter 1, I have broken down my recommendations for eating for fertility into three sections: what to eat, what not to eat, and how and when to eat. These provide a fairly comprehensive guide to good eating habits for fertility.

In addition, if you are dealing with PCOS:

- Choose foods that are low on the *glycemic index* (GI). The GI ranks foods according to the way they affect blood glucose levels. Check www.glycemicindex.com and the updated insulin index by Fiona McCulloch in *8 Steps to Reverse Your PCOS* for the most comprehensive food list available.[4]
- Avoid artificial sweeteners, as they increase inflammation and can negatively affect the growth of eggs.

A few other recommendations noted elsewhere are especially important for women with PCOS:

- Thirty minutes of daily exercise, such as brisk walking, dancing, or swimming, helps with weight loss and decreases sugar cravings. (Samantha chose to walk every day.)
- Exercises that build muscle strength, such as yoga or light weight-lifting, can help restore lean muscle mass; lean muscle tissue burns more sugar than fatty tissue, which helps reduce blood sugar and regulate insulin levels.
- Calming activities, such as meditation, yoga, Tai Chi, or Qi Gong, help soothe your spirit and lift your mood. (Samantha bought a DVD and did yoga at home twice a week.)

NOTE: If you are doing IVF, stop vigorous exercise during your IVF cycle, when there is potential for *ovarian hyperstimulation syndrome* (OHSS), a medical condition causing painful swelling in the ovaries as a result of excessive hormone stimulation. (See sidebar on page 119.)

Sleep your way to fertility

Sleep is important to all of us, but anyone who needs to regulate their blood sugar and insulin levels, especially in association with fertility, should make it a priority to get seven to nine hours of restful sleep every night. Chronically reducing sleep increases risk of metabolic disturbances that can lead to obesity and type 2 diabetes, which may cause ovulatory disturbances,[5] and waking up during the night to eat increases the risk of weight gain.[6]

Moreover, getting adequate sleep decreases sugar and caffeine cravings during the day. Indulging in sugar or caffeine when you are tired may give you a quick hit of energy, but it's typically followed by an energy low, which triggers cravings for more sugar and caffeine, and so on.

A regular sleeping pattern can also help regulate your reproductive hormones. You can support a good sleeping routine by:

- Going to sleep around the same time every night and waking up around the same time every morning. If you have a late night or poor sleep, take a twenty-minute nap in the afternoon to get you through the day without disrupting your sleep that night.
- Avoiding caffeine in the five to six hours before bedtime (or more, if you are sensitive to it).
- Avoiding alcohol, which disrupts sleep as soon as it wears off.
- Keeping your bedroom cool, dark, and quiet. Use blackout blinds or wear ear plugs if you have to, and make sure your bed and pillow are comfortable.[7]
- Relaxing before bed with a warm bath, calming music, or a guided meditation recording. If you read, avoid backlit e-books, which can stimulate your brain.
- Avoiding things that will stimulate you before bed, like working, exercising, watching TV, or having heated conversations. Don't go to bed mad or frustrated.
- Getting sunshine and fresh air during the day. It helps your body regulate your circadian rhythm (how well it is synchronized with external cues for sleep and wakefulness such as light and dark).

You can also take melatonin supplements. Melatonin is a hormone that helps regulate your body's circadian rhythm. People doing shift work or suffering jet lag sometimes take it as a supplement to help their body re-establish its circadian rhythm. It can support good IVF outcomes by triggering release of reproductive hormones and maintaining healthy egg and sperm development.

Preventing ovarian hyperstimulation syndrome

If you have a high AFC, you may run the risk of ovarian hyperstimulation syndrome (OHSS). OHSS is hyperstimulation of the ovaries in an attempt to make as many eggs as possible during IVF retrieval. The risk is that too many hormonal drugs can cause your ovaries to swell with an accumulation of fluid in the abdominal cavity.

In severe cases (twelve to fifteen percent)[8] it can lead to rapid weight gain, abdominal pain, vomiting, shortness of breath, development of blood clots, and compromise of kidney function (which occurs in five percent of the population even after pregnancy). This happened to one of my patients over a decade ago. It threatened her life, and, heartbreakingly, she had to terminate her pregnancy.

You can minimize the risk of OHSS naturally by:

- Drinking electrolyte drinks. Although Gatorade is considered the gold standard, it contains a lot of chemicals and sugar. You can make your own electrolyte drink or try coconut water.
- Eating salt. This is the only time I will ever tell you to eat chips and lots of them! Sodium and potassium are necessary as you lose sodium through the capillaries. Alternatively, take a teaspoon of sea salt daily.
- Eating protein. Protein helps form and prevent leaky blood capillaries, which contribute to OHSS.
- Avoiding exercise. Relax during stimulation. Since your ovaries are full, you'll likely feel too bloated and uncomfortable to exercise. Resting may also help you absorb the fluid in your abdomen by preventing capillaries from leaking during increased activity.
- Taking blood thinners. Low-dose aspirin may help prevent blood clots, as blood thickening can be a side effect of stimulation drugs and leaky capillaries.

Pre-conception acupuncture and Chinese herbal medicine

I recommend acupuncture once a week for four months and into the first trimester of pregnancy, and then monthly for pre-natal health. For PCOS, acupuncture relaxes the neuroendocrine system, which produces hormones, and can help to restore hormonal balance, ovulation, and menstruation.[9] Although Samantha had not had a period for five months, just two acupuncture sessions induced her flow. However, every individual is unique, which means response rate may vary.

Chinese herbal treatments work synergistically with acupuncture. Because herbal remedies are individually formulated, listing specific recommendations is beyond the scope of this book. I recommend consulting a TCM practitioner who works with fertility issues. If you are working with a TCM herbalist, be up front and ask if they are taking precautionary measures in sourcing uncontaminated herbs. Consider it a red flag if they do not know where their distributor obtains their herbs.

Samantha's spark of life

While she was off work, Samantha found another job through a friend's recommendation. She later told me she did not realize how much stress she'd been living with until she started working in a supportive environment.

I often see patients who aren't aware of how much stress they are under until they are away from it. It's the body's coping mechanism. But the body works very differently in survival mode than in what I call "thrival" mode. Your body might be giving you signals that you are just surviving, like headaches, insomnia, weight gain, emotional anxiety, stress, tension, or irregular menstruation. Be kind to yourself. Pay attention when your body asks for what it needs.

At Samantha's new workplace, her manager told her about a friend who did IVF. This gave Samantha an opportunity to share her fertility issues. Her boss was empathetic, and instead of tracking her time at work, she told her to take her time, as long as the work got done.

Samantha's periods came back naturally and she conceived shortly after that in the comfort of her own home. She continued with acupuncture during the first trimester. Her conception was not the result of one specific thing but the myriad ways in which Samantha had changed her life, allowing her to create a little spark named Isabella.

Sally: Endometriosis

Sally was thirty-four years old when she came to me. She'd been married for seven years and trying to conceive for four years, on and off. Although she had regular menstrual cycles, she had *endometriosis*, a condition that can cause severe pain in the pelvis as tissues that normally reside in the uterus, the *endometrium*, grow outside the uterus. She'd had three *laparoscopic* surgeries over six years. The first two, when she was twenty-four and twenty-seven, were to deal with severe pain. After her second surgery, she became vegan, following an anti-inflammatory, plant-based diet. The primary goal of her third surgery, at thirty, was to remove endometrial tissue around her bowels and ovaries and *endometriomas* (hormone-dependent ovarian cysts), a plausible cause for her fertility challenges.

Sally was a researcher who was working two jobs and completing her PhD. A frequent lecturer and presenter, she often worked countless hours with tight deadlines. As if a busy work schedule and trying to conceive with painful endometriosis were not stressful enough, she and her husband had been dealing with family health crises, which had caused them to put baby-making on the back burner. First, her mother-in-law had died of cancer, and then her father had a heart attack. After this, Sally and her husband had gone to a fertility doctor and she'd gone through two non-medicated rounds of cycle monitoring with timed intercourse, followed by two medicated rounds of IUI, with no baby to show for her efforts.

Sally had never had acupuncture but wanted to try something outside of conventional medicine, as she was not keen to go through another surgery for endometriosis. When she came to see me, she had fibroids and pelvic adhesions on her left ovary and chronic low back pain.

Recognizing her stress levels, I asked who in her life knew she was having difficulty conceiving. She'd confided only in her best friend and her mother. In fact, most people assumed she and her husband didn't want children because they were focused on their careers. I suggested that she share her fertility issues with someone at work that she could trust. Perhaps she could negotiate a different work structure to decrease her stress and create a work environment more conducive to baby-making.

She was already in the middle of her third IUI cycle when she came to me, but she started taking herbal medicine and having acupuncture weekly. Because she really wanted a baby, she took my advice and made life-altering changes, which included cutting out coffee and alcohol. She also toned down her usually vigorous exercise routine to allow more energy and blood to flow to her reproductive organs. For example, rather than running ten or twenty kilometres, she went for five-kilometre runs or long brisk walks, which helped her connect with nature and de-stress.

Sally also took my recommendation to change her work habits. She started by letting her manager know she was going to the fertility clinic in the mornings and doing weekly acupuncture treatments in an effort to have a baby. With her manager's support, she worked two days from home to lessen her stress.

By getting her body out of fight-or-flight mode, she created an environment conducive to allowing energy to flow freely to her reproductive organs, increasing her chances of conception.

Increasing blood flow to reproductive organs

FEMORAL ARTERY MASSAGE

Femoral massage is a self-massage that you or your partner can do in the comfort of your own home daily from menses to ovulation. Or if you are preparing for an IVF embryo transfer, you can do it up until transfer day but not after the transfer. The point is to increase energy and blood flow to your reproductive organs.[10]

The femoral artery is a blood vessel that feeds your legs. It branches off the main (iliac) artery in the trunk of your body; one branch feeds the femoral artery and the other supplies the internal organs. When you press on the femoral artery, more blood flows to your internal organs than your legs.

You can find your femoral artery by putting your index and middle fingers together in your groin (where your leg crease is) and feeling for a pulse located about one-third of the way from the inside of the thigh to the outside. Press on this pulse point for thirty seconds to briefly redirect blood to your ovaries, fallopian tubes, and uterus. Then do it on your other leg for thirty seconds. Repeat three times per leg, and do this twice daily.

Note: Do not do this if you are pregnant, or think you might be, have a history of blood clots, or have a circulatory disorder, heart disease, high blood pressure, or detached retinas.

CASTOR OIL PACK

You can buy castor oil at the health food store or most pharmacies. Put one cup in a microwavable plastic container. Cut out an old piece of flannel, large enough to cover the area from your hip bones to the top of your pubic bone, and just under your navel. Put the flannel into the container of castor oil and heat it for twenty seconds. Wring it out lightly, then place it on your tummy, just under the belly button. Cover it with a piece of plastic cling wrap, and then put on an old t-shirt on top of this. Heat up a microwavable grain bag (or use a hot water bottle) and put it on top of the t-shirt and over the flannel area. Keep it on for thirty minutes in the evenings and relax. Doing this daily from the end of your period to ovulation increases blood flow to the ovaries and uterus, carrying nutrients and oxygen that help to break up old adhesions and fibroids.

Note: Do not do this after ovulation, if you are pregnant or breastfeeding, or if you have an open wound.

HOT EPSOM SALTS FOOT BATH
Find a foot bath (any plastic container that can fit your feet will do). Fill with hot water and add a half-cup of Epsom salts. Sit on a comfortable chair, close your eyes, and soak your feet for fifteen minutes to increase circulation and induce a relaxation response.

Workplace strategies for conception

Unfortunately for Samantha, the workplace is not always supportive of employees dealing with fertility challenges. Yet this is poor business sense. Even though no one talks about it at work, statistically, if you have eighteen people in a board meeting, three of them are having, have had, or will have fertility issues in their lifetime.[11] Educating your employer about fertility challenges and the demands of using a fertility clinic will help your workplace become more supportive to employees, which is likely to increase their loyalty and effectiveness, as opposed to failing to support them and converting a dedicated worker like Samantha into an unhappy, disgruntled, resentful, and unmotivated employee looking for a way out.

Sally, however, was able to build support in her workplace to make it more conducive to creating a baby. The following are some of the strategies you can try to make your workplace less stressful. If these aren't effective where you work, they at least provide you with an idea of the kind of workplace to look for:

- Create a supportive community. Find someone at work you can trust—a colleague, a manager, or a human resources officer—and talk to them about your difficulties conceiving.
- Ask to work flexible shifts. The ability to come in later and work later can decrease your stress about getting to work at a specific time when you are not sure what time you will be done at the fertility clinic daily.[12]
- Suggest part-time telecommuting. Working from home several times weekly reduces commute time, eliminates coffee break chatter, and promotes more efficiency and effectiveness so you can get your job done in less time (and also get to your medical appointments or focus on de-stressing activities like yoga or long walks in between).
- Minimize extra workload and speaking engagements. There will be times in your career for proving yourself at work. This is not one of them. This is the time to work smarter, not harder.
- Minimize work travel. If your work involves a lot of travel, consider giving an opportunity to a colleague. Travel increases stress when you are timing intercourse at ovulation, or needing to be monitored at a fertility clinic in preparation for IUI or IVF.

Even if you do not feel you can talk to anyone at your workplace about your fertility challenges, you can still request flexible shifts and telecommuting options one or two days each week.

Data from the US National Study of the Changing Workforce found that flexible work times help reduce overall stress and foster higher levels of commitment to employers.[13] Working from home can reduce organizational costs by reducing both absenteeism and missed deadlines. In the end, changes like these can be a win-win for you and your employer.

Sally's "little fire" baby

Three months after Sally began working with me, with the help of a low-dose injectable hormone stimulant called Puragon on her fourth IUI cycle, she became pregnant. Unlike Samantha, she did not have to leave an unsupportive workplace to make it happen. In fact, the month she conceived was her busiest time at work.

Sally could not pinpoint one thing that had worked. She had been eating right and exercising moderately as a means to decompress. She had been getting acupuncture in an environment she described as a sanctuary compared to the sterile atmosphere of the fertility clinic. She had also been creating more supportive home and work environments.

In short, she had combined the best of Eastern and Western medicine. For her, the warmth and comfort of acupuncture and TCM had offset the stressfulness of the fertility clinic treatments. This had improved the physical and emotional balance in her life, which not only helped her conceive but supported her in bringing her healthy "little fire" baby, Ethan, into this world naturally.

7

Making the Impossible Possible

Natural forces within us are the true healers of disease.

HIPPOCRATES

Miriam: Autoimmune infertility

Miriam, a banker, met her husband at nineteen. They married at thirty-two, and she got pregnant accidentally but miscarried. They didn't investigate the cause of the miscarriage and continued using contraception until they decided to focus on building a family when Miriam was thirty-four. Despite the miscarriage, she did not anticipate any problems and certainly did not expect a seven-year journey.

When they did not get pregnant after one year, they went to a fertility clinic, and she was diagnosed with unexplained infertility. She underwent four IVF cycles prior to coming to my clinic on the recommendation of a friend. At this point, frustrated by a diagnosis that provided no explanations for her failed IVFs, and therefore without a treatment strategy, Miriam was experiencing anxiety and depression. She sought TCM treatments to balance her body before undergoing any more procedures with the fertility clinic.

After working together for two months, she was thrilled to conceive twins with her fifth IVF, but her joy quickly turned to devastation when an ultrasound revealed they'd stopped developing at six weeks. Miriam had a D&C and the products of conception were analyzed, revealing an unexpected genetic issue called *Robertsonian translocation*, in which a piece of a chromosome breaks off and is moved onto another chromosome, resulting in structural chromosomal abnormalities.

Now, in addition to feeling reproductively "old," Miriam was dealing with a genetic issue. Fortunately, it could be addressed by doing IVF with pre-implantation genetic screening (PGS), a process of removing one cell from a day five or six embryo, which has many cells. The embryo is then tested for genetic viability before being transferred to the uterus.

Chromosomal translocation

This condition accounts for two to four percent of recurrent pregnancy losses.[1] According to a study out of the Netherlands, couples in which one is a carrier are twenty percent more at risk of miscarriages over non-carrier couples experiencing recurrent miscarriage. In both cases, they are equally likely to give birth to a healthy child.

Normally, women are only tested for chromosomal translocation issues after two or more miscarriages. Men can have the same chromosomal abnormality causing miscarriage. About one person in 500 has a balanced translocation, which makes it uncommon, as documented in 1998.[2] One study showed that only 0.1 percent of 1415 (Japanese) couples (two women out of 1415) experiencing multiple miscarriages had translocation mutations.[3]

Chromosomal balanced translocations or rearrangements can happen naturally during sperm production (especially in older men) or when the sperm unites with egg at fertilization. They may develop spontaneously or be passed down in families from parent to child. This chromosomal rearrangement can occur "irrelevant to men's lifestyle, environment or work."[4]

Intensive intervention

Miriam's problems didn't end there. She also had *uterine fibroids,* which are non-cancerous tumors composed of dense, fibrous tissue. Although they'd been present for as long as I'd been seeing her, upon examination after the D&C, I noticed they'd grown to the point that they were visibly distending her abdomen. Chinese medicine and acupuncture can help dissipate or shrink fibroids up to about three centimetres, but if they are longstanding and dense, they are unlikely to be eliminated naturally. Miriam's fibroids were not seen as a factor in her fertility challenges. That is because many women who have fibroids do not experience impaired ability to get and stay pregnant.

Having been exposed to multiple rounds of IVF and due to her twin pregnancy, Miriam had a surplus of hormones in her body, which had likely fuelled the growth of her fibroids. When they became palpable by hand, I explained that they could be another factor interfering with embryo implantation and development, and Miriam requested that her fertility doctor perform a *myomectomy*, a surgical procedure to remove them, before trying another round of IVF. During the procedure, the doctor removed nineteen fibroids, ranging in size from marbles to tennis balls.

What is autoimmune infertility?

Miriam continued to relentlessly search for answers to her failed pregnancies, suspecting she had immune issues because her mother had *Sjogren's disease* (dry eyes and mouth as a result of immune cells interfering with salivary and tear gland secretions) and her sister had hypothyroidism. Miriam paid for extensive testing by the controversial Alan Beer Resource Centre for Reproductive Immunology and Genetics, which offers treatments not approved by most fertility clinics (including Miriam's). She was diagnosed with autoimmune infertility, meaning her immune system was rejecting the embryo or preventing implantation.

Controversial treatments

Typically, Western medical fertility specialists believe some women's immune systems recognize and reject their partner's or donor sperm, or embryos, as "foreign" invaders. The immune system protects the woman from this foreign invader by preventing fertilization, implantation, or development during pregnancy. This can lead to repeated failed IVF attempts or recurrent miscarriages.

Dr. Alan Beer, author of *Is Your Body Baby Friendly?*,[5] has developed some controversial treatments to treat fertility challenges related to an autoimmune response. Some women with complex fertility challenges have successfully used some of these treatments to carry a healthy baby to term. But the treatments are controversial because they use blood by-products made from up to 50,000 healthy donors mixed together, which are then injected into the woman as a therapy.

Miriam opted for a treatment called *lymphocyte immunization therapy* (LIT), which involves injecting the male partner's washed and extracted white blood cells into the female's forearm.[6] Theoretically, this allows the body's immune system to develop an antibody response to her partner's cells so her immune system will recognize the embryo as "self" rather than an invader to be killed off. As of 2016, this treatment is illegal in the United States and only offered in Canada to patients at Markham Fertility Centre (just outside of Toronto).

At the time Miriam did LIT, it was not available in Canada, so she and her husband went to great lengths to have it performed in Mexico. First, they drove to a Macdonald's on the American side of the U.S./Mexico border, where a van transported them to a lab on the Mexican side. It was a weird and sketchy experience, but the only side effect of the treatment was itching at the injection site. Like most patients, Miriam did multiple treatments in preparation for IVF. Once the patient becomes pregnant, she gets booster shots every five to seven weeks to protect the baby. I can only imagine how stressful and costly it must have been for them to travel to Mexico for this treatment every time.

In addition, Miriam had intravenous immunoglobulin G (IVIg) treatments.[7] Theoretically, this IV drip cocktail of immune cells (antibodies), again from the blood products of up to 50,000 donors, prevents damage to the embryo and uterine cells as a result of an abnormal immune response. Specifically, it aims to decrease excessively high levels of Natural Killer (NK) cells from attacking the partners' sperm or the embryo.

Finally, Miriam took Dexamethasone (a steroid) and Fragmin (a blood thinner) throughout her IVF treatments. The steroid was used to reduce inflammation and autoimmune response by reducing NK cell activity. Although this was not Miriam's issue, it can also decrease male hormones like testosterone, which can contribute to PCOS. The blood thinner was to prevent blood clot formation, which can cause miscarriage. These two drugs are standard treatments that her fertility clinic advised her to undertake for autoimmune issues.

As for having LIT and IVIg treatments, Miriam opted not to tell her fertility clinic while undergoing IVF with them, because she knew her doctor did not approve of them. This added to her stress at a time when stress was the last thing her body needed.

My view on autoimmune infertility

Alan Beer, the inventor of the controversial procedures described above (among others), believed a woman's activated immune system could damage the placenta or embryo, reject implantation, or interfere with reproductive hormones and prevent pregnancy from occurring. Correcting this required immunosuppressive treatment so the woman's body would recognize that embryos were not foreign invaders. In describing this phenomenon, he wrote, "women become serial killers to their own babies."[8] I find this harsh, judgmental, and blaming, as if the woman with an autoimmune reaction is at fault.

I see autoimmune reactions as the body's way of expressing its state of being out of balance, but thinking it's doing the right thing, and protecting itself from harm. While I've had patients like Miriam who've used Beer's strategies to become pregnant, and I am not opposed to such treatment, from a TCM standpoint, it's a symptomatic treatment in that it does not address the underlying cause of the autoimmune reaction.

TCM would ask why your body is seeing an embryo as a foreign invader in the first place. Perhaps it's another way your body says, "No, not now" to having a baby. With blood tests showing excessive antibodies, NK cells, and other autoimmune markers, this might be a sign that your body is reacting to prolonged internal and external environmental stressors. Perhaps supporting this theory, Miriam did not have to do the autoimmune protocols for her second pregnancy. Neither Did Krista, my second autoimmune case study. I will tell her story later in this chapter.

It's stressful to think your own immune system is like an army of soldiers killing off your embryos. And negative thinking can contribute to creating an unappealing environment for a baby to move into. When my patients have autoimmune challenges, I encourage them to think about what's happening in their lives that could give their body a reason to say no to having a baby right now. I urge them not to self-blame but to reflect about what is not aligned within themselves at the present time or in the past, and to ask when they last experienced peace, happiness, love, or connectedness. This diagnosis is not a question of whether you deserve to get pregnant, and it certainly is not your fault. It is simply a state of being at a moment in time. Under the right conditions, your immune response may be normalized.

Everything but the kitchen sink

Miriam was resourceful in taking control of her fertility health and trying just about everything a woman can do to have a child in her womb. In addition to IVF treatments with genetic testing, paired with travelling to undergo immunosuppressive treatments, she kept working at a full-time job. She came to my clinic regularly for acupuncture, she did yoga and meditated, she had Mayan abdominal massage (a special massage for increasing blood flow to the reproductive organs while trying to break up any scar tissue or inflammation), and she tried hypnosis, energy healing, and colonic irrigation.

She took supplements including CoQ10 and PQQ to help with egg quality (see Chapter 4), fish oil to decrease inflammation, milk thistle to support detoxification, and wheatgrass to clear out excess hormones from previous IVFs. She took Chinese herbs to move internal static blood and decrease inflammation, as well as DHEA, an adrenal hormone that converts to testosterone or estrogen and is thought to enhance egg quality. Upon my suggestion, she switched to an organic gluten- and dairy-free diet. Finally, she went to a naturopathic doctor, who tested her for food allergies and removed certain foods from her diet that, according to her blood tests, triggered an immune response.

From a Western perspective, Miriam had a complex set of fertility challenges from unexplained to autoimmune infertility, with genetic factors, fibroids, and advanced maternal age thrown in. When she conceived following IVF with PGS prior to frozen embryo transfer (FET, in which embryos harvested during a previous IVF cycle are frozen and then thawed before transfer to the uterus), anyone might have said it was these interventions, as well as the immunosuppressive therapy, that enabled her to conceive and carry beautiful baby Audrey to term.

However, from a TCM perspective, while these treatments addressed her symptoms, they also caused side effects that threw her body even more out of balance. Specifically, her fibroids grew to the point she needed to have them surgically removed, and the stress of the whole process may have increased her body's immune response.

After the many years I've worked with women who defy the odds and become pregnant, I believe TCM, lifestyle and dietary changes, and positive thoughts are as important as technological interventions. And perhaps these things helped Miriam maintain as much balance as possible while pursuing extreme treatments, and benefitted her in ways science does not yet comprehend.

One more time

Although Miriam was grateful for baby Audrey, she kept thinking that she had one chromosomally normal embryo sitting on ice. She and her husband wanted to try for a second child. She came back to me for some acupuncture treatments to help rebalance her body before she attempted another FET, which I like to describe as picking up the kid from the skating rink.

Miriam was maintaining her healthy diet and resumed her pre-conception treatments, focusing her attention on creating a healthy environment, toxin-free and populated with positive thoughts, feelings, and expectations. As well, her recent auto-immune testing indicated that her body was no longer in an overactive immune state—it was no longer saying, "no, not now." I agreed with Miriam that it seemed like her body was receptive, and she went ahead with a transfer, using her final frozen embryo. As I write, she has just given birth to her second child, Thomas, via C-section. Thankfully, all went smoothly and they are just adjusting to demanding newborn schedules of eating and sleeping every two hours.

Epigenetics

This is where the science of epigenetics comes in, where gene expression and appearance can be turned on or off, and even passed down to your children, depending on internal and external environments. That means your DNA does not have the final word in determining your genetics.

Dr. Bruce Lipton, author of *The Biology of Belief*,[9] states that a "cell's life is controlled by the physical and energetic environment and not by its genes." That means what we think, believe, and perceive can impact our brain in releasing a cascade of hormones that can ultimately affect our reproductive function, egg cell division, egg development, and uterine lining. That is, how we respond to our environment physically, mental, emotionally, and spiritually affects our health and, in this case, our fertility.

Dr. Lipton goes on to say that "beliefs control biology." According to him, by being conscious and aware of our thoughts and perceptions of things, events, and stresses in our lives and then altering our responses to them, we can impact our brain chemistry, which then impacts everything down to the way our cells grow, divide, and thrive. As he puts it, "we are not stuck with our genes or our self-defeating behaviours!"[10]

Western medicine, he says, "fixes" the body like a mechanic fixes a car in terms of its parts. But what about the driver? It's not the mechanic's job to fix both car and driver, but it is arguably the doctor's job to do so.

Back to Chinese medicine

Dr. Lipton's ideas about epigenetics are in line with the beliefs underlying Chinese medicine. All imbalances and disease are due to external and internal etiologies. External causes of illness relate to your exposure to your environment, toxins, how and what you eat and do in life, and what things happen to you (like physical trauma). Internal causes of illness stem from the seven affects of emotions introduced in Chapter 2: sadness, anger, worry, grief, fear, fright (shock), and anxiety experienced in excess for prolonged periods of time. In modern times, you can understand it in terms of the mind/body connection. What and how we think and feel can affect the 50 trillion cells in our bodies, the largest of which is a woman's egg.

Although we may not be able to change everything in our environment or life circumstances, we can to some extent alter the way we think about them and respond to them, which can impact our bodies right down to our DNA. So how do we do that? TCM encourages us to nourish our bodies and decrease inflammation and stagnation of blood and energy with specific herbs. Acupuncture helps to increase serotonin and endorphin output, and improve the cascade of hormones that stimulate ovulation[11] and regulate immune function.[12]

If the immune system, a physical system, breaks down, it can mess up the way our bodies respond to pathogens, or it can cause our bodies to perceive invaders where there are none. If we retain energy by repressing emotions over a long period of time, we can deprive our bodies of the energy they need to function properly.

Bringing our bodies back into balance includes correcting dietary and lifestyle choices by eating better (see Chapter 1: Eating for fertility), getting moderate exercise, and sleeping adequately, as well as minimizing exposure to environmental pollutants, toxins, amalgam fillings (mercury), contaminated foods, chemically laden foods, pesticides, and overuse of antibiotics.

Bringing our bodies back into balance also includes recognizing that, because we are constantly bombarded with toxins, it's easy for our livers, which exist to filter toxins out of our bodies, to become overworked, and wise to support this organ to clear out accumulated toxicity.

In TCM, we also believe the liver can become overworked by trying to dispel emotional toxins. Emotions that get stuck internally, like the unfulfilled desire to have a baby, and the anguish, sadness, grief, worry, and fear that go along with that, can cause the liver to get stuck energetically, negatively impacting its physical function.

We can prevent emotional toxins from building up by consciously changing the way we respond to situations. For example, the next time you go to a dinner party with girlfriends you have not seen in a long time, and there is a lot of baby talk, remind yourself it's likely one of them had fertility issues, and use that as hope. And if that doesn't work, sit beside someone who does not have children and engage in different conversation. Then again, if you know that you are not up for the social interaction, do not feel guilty or force yourself to go but, instead, graciously opt out of going to dinner.

Although it's best to see a TCM practitioner for help in determining your particular problems and detoxifying your liver, you can help it somewhat on your own by drinking hot lemon water, dandelion leaf tea, and peppermint tea, and taking chlorella, wheat grass, and Chinese liver cleansing herbs, like dandelion leaves (Pu Gong Ying), chrysanthemum (Ju Hua), and honeysuckle (Jin Yin Hua).

Other autoimmune disorders

Having an autoimmune disorder like lupus or rheumatoid arthritis does not automatically mean you will have fertility issues. I have seen women with both these issues maintain their overall balance and well-being, conceive quickly, and have healthy babies without a hitch. For example, Vanessa in Chapter 1 had rheumatoid arthritis. Although she initially had difficulty conceiving, she ended up naturally conceiving her two kids.

You can't force positivity

You hear it all the time: just think positive. But it's not that simple.

On the premise that what you think and believe can ultimately impact cells and gene expression, I am not telling you to just "think positive." That might just make you sick to your stomach. Forcing yourself to think positive is like putting icing on a mud pie. It's inauthentic.

If you were to think only positive thoughts when you're going through a difficult time, all you'd be doing is suppressing the feelings of sadness, anger, grief, fear, worry, and frustration, which can be locked deep within your subconscious mind. And these subconscious thoughts, emotions, and beliefs are most likely to impact your cells and genes. Harbouring negative emotions over prolonged periods requires energy, which means you could be investing a considerable amount of your body's energy in shoving your feelings down. This can deplete your overall energy and put you back into fight-or-flight mode. So give yourself permission to let go, to feel and embrace your thoughts and emotions, even when doing so feels difficult and uncomfortable.

The art of letting go

Your subconscious thoughts create a certain "truth" or "reality" in your life. At least, you believe it's the "truth," and you have specific emotions directly associated with this subconscious belief.

In a nutshell, what you suppress emotionally is directly associated with your beliefs. This resides in your subconscious mind and is more powerful than your conscious mind by a long shot. As Dr. Lipton said in an interview,[13] we "operate ninety-five to ninety-nine percent of our lives from subconscious programs."

The negative energy generated by your beliefs gets ingrained all the way down to your cells. Your subconscious belief that "My eggs are too old" or "It's impossible for me to have a baby" and the emotional devastation that accompanies this belief can have a powerful negative impact on your cells.

The good news is that you can reprogram your subconscious beliefs and let them go. And once reprogrammed, healing can take place and your cells can respond differently. Different types of therapies can help you heal, such as hypnosis, meditation, and several psychology therapies, including emotional freedom technique (EFT), cognitive behavioural therapy (CBT), and eye movement desensitization and reprocessing (EMDR), to name a few. In a powerful example, one study looked at the effects of hypnosis on embryo transfer in IVF and showed it to double pregnancy rates compared to a control group of women who did not do hypnosis.[14]

The three Rs of positive self-talk

Positive self-talk is not about persuading yourself to be positive. Rather, it is a technique to help you visualize positive images to replace the negative images stuck deep in your subconscious mind. The three Rs of positive self-talk is a simple technique used by Shawn Gallagher, the hypnofertility practitioner at our clinic, to help let go of your internal beliefs, stop the stress-in-fertility-stress cycle, and enhance your fertility:

- RECOGNIZE in your self-talk what thoughts do not support success. This first step is essential: you cannot change what you are unaware of.
- RELEASE non-supportive thoughts. A simple way to do this is to imagine a big cancel/delete button in your mind and send it to a virtual trash box. Many of us have thoughts that replay over and over, and sometimes we feel powerless when that hamster wheel in the mind is spinning. But we can take control.
- REPLACE these thoughts with positive statements and images that provide clear direction for your mind.

For example, perhaps your negative belief is that your eggs are too old. First, you need to recognize that tape playing over and over in your mind. Second, you need to release that; there are many ways of visualizing this, but let's assume you're sending it to the virtual trash in your brain. Third, you need to replace that negative tape with something positive, like "I'm surrounding my ovaries with healing energy." At the same time, you might also want to imagine your ovaries soaking up all that good energy and creating healthy, happy follicles that mature into beautiful eggs.

Here's one of the easiest ways to incorporate the three Rs throughout your day: If a negative thought pops into your mind, take a few seconds to practice recognizing the thought, releasing it, and replacing it with a positive statement or image before continuing with your usual activities.

If you can find a few moments of quiet, get comfortable, take a few slow deep breaths, centre yourself, and focus on a positive statement. You can repeat a statement in your mind only, but verbalizing aloud helps re-pattern additional brain functions. Initially, this can feel awkward, but it gets easier with practice.

Positive statements and images speak the language of the inner mind. As you reinforce your mind in positive ways, whether through the three Rs, meditation, or a therapy such as CBT, you may find your TCM treatments becoming more effective and longer-lasting.

Positive self-talk is also an essential component of self-hypnosis. The inner mind has a limited ability to understand negations. If I tell you not to think about an elephant, your inner mind ignores the "not" and calls up pictures and stories of elephants. Releasing a non-supportive thought and replacing it with one that focuses on your goal is a way for your conscious mind to influence your inner mind.[15]

In Deepak Chopra's book *Unconditional Life: Discovering the Power to Fulfill Your Dreams*, he writes, "the fleeting, invisible impulses of the mind can turn into concrete, locatable neurotransmitter molecules like dopamine and serotonin."[16] In other words, your thoughts and emotions create a physical impact in your body. Positive self-talk can impact your body and your cells in a positive way.

Positive thoughts to support fertility healing

You may find it helpful to recognize your most frequently recurring negative thoughts and write your replace statements on index cards or post them in your home, car, or workplace as frequent reminders to repeat them to yourself. You can also be digitally creative by adding them to your calendar, phone, or computer screen.

Some people also find it helpful to have a buddy system, where a partner or friend can gently remind you to hit the cancel/delete button and use one of your replace statements instead. Here are some replace statements you might use or adapt to your needs:

- I surround my ovaries, tubes, and uterus with healing energy and love.
- My body easily creates healthy, perfect eggs.
- My body ovulates at the perfect time, in the perfect way for an easy pregnancy.
- I choose healthy, nutritious food to support an easy pregnancy to term.
- I open my heart to my baby or babies.
- My hormone levels are healthy, balanced, and strong,
- I fill my uterus with love and happiness.
- My pregnancy is safe and healthy all the way to term.

Most people find the "replace" part of the three Rs to be the biggest challenge. For many of us initially, a statement that's believable is more important than one that's positive. Making too big a jump from negative to positive usually sets up resistance, and can make us feel more miserable because it highlights that what we want hasn't happened yet. Eventually, you will learn to ease yourself into a state of happier anticipation. With time, positive internal dialogue will become natural and automatic.

Krista: PCOS and autoimmune infertility

Krista started trying to conceive when she was thirty-one. At a young age, she'd complained of irregular periods and her doctor had discovered she did not always ovulate. At eighteen, she was diagnosed with polycystic ovarian syndrome (PCOS) and was told it would be difficult for her to conceive. Imagine how devastating that must have been at such a young age.

This was a source of anxiety for her, both because she had depressive tendencies to begin with and because she knew even then that she wanted children. For thirteen years, she carried the belief that she could not have a baby naturally, and stored her emotions of grief, fear, and worry deep inside her.

When she came to see me, she had been trying to conceive for six months and was already at a fertility clinic. She had a thin endometrial lining and erratic menses, where she had a period every thirty-five-plus days. She had two days of menstrual pain, had acne, and had never been pregnant. Being the daughter of a physician, she took statistics and numbers to heart and always anticipated the worst possible outcome.

Complicating matters, her husband had male factor infertility (MFI) with poor sperm morphology, motility, and count. Thankfully, that was remedied through the use of vitamins (see Chapter 5 for a list of recommended vitamins), and his sperm count increased from 19 million per cc to 75 million. Meanwhile, Krista had acupuncture and took herbal medicine and lots of supplements. Miraculously, because she'd believed it to be impossible, she became pregnant after eight months of trying. Sadly, she miscarried.

Now she was not only stressed by the possibility of being unable to conceive but, if she did, being unable to carry a baby to term. And when she looked at the many written lab results month after a month, all she saw was that her reproductive hormones were out of whack—she had an abnormally high LH:FSH ratio (luteinizing hormone to follicle stimulating hormone), which is consistent with PCOS.

Always looking for pathology, she went to a doctor for immune testing. More lab findings showed she had low

T-Regulatory cells (which keep the immune system in check so it doesn't kill everything off), low leukocyte antibodies, elevated anti-lupus anticoagulant antibodies, anti-sperm antibodies, MTHFR heterozygous gene mutation, and clotting factor. Basically, that's a lot of big words that point to autoimmune infertility issues. Like Miriam, Krista was advised to do LIT, but as it was such a controversial treatment, she did not feel comfortable with it.

I told her I did not have all the answers and couldn't guarantee anything. However, I could see that she was under constant stress trying to overcome her fertility challenges. I told her that focusing on acronyms, lab numbers, and statistics was overwhelming her, which could be exacerbating the imbalance in her body. I suggested that instead of focusing on pregnancy, with an outcome she could not control, she might focus on the little things in her life like what and how she ate, and how to decrease her daily stress levels.

She told me that she loved kids and she loved being an elementary school teacher but she found work very stressful. Instead of feeling fulfilled by her work, it was taking a toll on her health because her principal was not supportive of her predicament. Making matters worse, trips to the fertility doctor became challenging as she had no control over the length of her appointments and would often arrive at school late, which did not go well in that non-supportive environment.

Krista's little miracle

Krista's story exemplifies the role of epigenetics, showing how her thoughts and beliefs were quite possibly impacting the cells in her body. But being proactive with acupuncture, Chinese herbs, and supplements, and slowly watching her menstrual cycle change, provided the evidence she needed to feel more confident that she could overcome her condition and get pregnant. Within four months of beginning treatments, Krista's anti-sperm antibodies had decreased dramatically, while her T-Regulatory cells had increased.

And then she decided to take back some control in her life and submitted her letter of resignation for the end of the school term. This took a huge weight off her back. A month after giving her notice, seven months after her first miscarriage, she was pregnant. This time, she carried the baby to term and recently gave birth to her miracle daughter, Olivia, weighing in at a petite but healthy six pounds, seven ounces.

The moral of this story

Remember: the impossible can be possible. You are more than just a set of lab values, even when they look like they are permanent. Do not let your diagnosis define who you are and what you are capable of. Instead, consider it a baseline marker and an opportunity to change how you live your life.

You can heal yourself by working on the physical level (lifestyle, dietary habits, treatments like acupuncture and hypnosis) and, equally important, on the mental, emotional, and spiritual levels (such as finding peace in the moment, as Krista did by leaving her toxic workplace). Align your life in order to create life. Alter things you can control rather than focusing on things you cannot control.

To date, there is no treatment to fix chromosomal or genetic defects. IVF with PGS testing of embryos can minimize the chances of a non-viable pregnancy leading to miscarriage, but it is not foolproof. Even when the results come back that an embryo is genetically perfect, they do not guarantee a pregnancy.

Science may look for the underlying pathology when things don't work, but we cannot always quantify such things. Nor can we always explain when life's miracles happen. But they do. Just ask Miriam and Krista. They both had everything but the kitchen sink going against them, yet they both conceived and carried their beautiful little miracles to term.

8

"This Can't Be Happening to Me"

Only the wounded physician heals.

CARL JUNG

Mary: Blocked fallopian tubes

"Why the hell can't I get pregnant?" I asked myself numerous times every day. I was happy and led a healthy life: I ate organic food, I didn't smoke, I didn't drink coffee or alcohol. I prided myself on never getting sick. Both of my grandmothers had children at age forty-six. I should have been a fertility goddess, but instead, I found myself struggling to conceive when I was ready to have a family at thirty-eight.

Adding insult to injury, I am a registered TCM practitioner and I work with women who have fertility challenges every day. I'd helped countless women and couples to conceive. I felt like a fraud being unable to get pregnant myself.

"It must be his fault"

At first, I was convinced my husband's beer- and wine-drinking habits were the root cause of our infertility. After all, alcohol can be associated with a decrease in normal sperm formation.

But Jean-Louis's tests indicated he had a stellar sperm count of over 100 million per millilitre, 20 million being the low end of the "normal." Sperm-wise, he was a proud and virile superstar, yet I was secretly disappointed because it meant our problems were my problems.

After months of testing, my second fertility doctor confirmed that both of my fallopian tubes were blocked and fluid-filled, a condition called *bilateral hydrosalpinx*. To my dismay, this was one condition I'd had little success with in my own practice. Think of it this way: the tubes are as thin as dental floss. This condition can heal if it has not been long standing and the fallopian tubes are not yet distorted, but mine were too far gone. Under the *hysterosalpingogram*, an x-ray where they shoot a dye into the vagina, I saw the tortuous (crooked and twisted) tubes. It felt like a cruel, cosmic joke that, seemingly overnight, I'd joined the ranks of the many women who came to my clinic for help.

What are blocked fallopian tubes?

The fallopian tubes are two tubes from the uterus that catch the egg from the ovary upon ovulation. Sperm swim up the fallopian tubes to fertilize the egg.

Blockage of one tube reduces chances of pregnancy by fifty percent. If both tubes are blocked then there is no chance of pregnancy. They can be blocked by *adhesions* (where scar tissues connects things that are not normally connected) or by fluid (hydrosalpinx). Causes for tubal blockages include:

- Biological abnormality at birth.
- Occlusions from polyps or fibroids that develop right at the entryway from the uterus to fallopian tube(s).
- Ectopic pregnancy, where conception takes place in the fallopian tubes. Such pregnancies become non-viable and

are sometimes removed surgically or resolved with medication, which can leave behind scar tissue in the affected tube; other times, the whole tube is removed, leaving the woman with only one tube.

- Other pelvic surgery leaving behind scar tissues and adhesions.
- Peritonitis, which is a potentially serious, even fatal, inflammation of the lining of the abdominal cavity.
- Pelvic infections or STI, the most prevalent of which is chlamydia, a bacterial infection that is often asymptomatic and can be undetected for years.
- Endometriosis, which, when severe, can cause endometrial tissue and scar tissue to block the tubes.

Basically, STI can be caught quickly if a woman has regular Pap smears (where a speculum is inserted into the cervix and then swabbed and tested for cervical cancer and other diseases). Catching STI quickly and treating them with strong antibiotics can prevent the spread and severity of pelvic infections and inflammation, and prevent tubal blockages from developing. However, if left untreated and with the passage of time, infection and inflammation can severely damage the fallopian tubes, leaving scar tissues that will eventually become irreparable. This often occurs without any symptoms. If the tubes become fluid-filled, the fluids can be toxic to implantation. In this case, the only treatment is laparoscopic micro-surgical removal of the fallopian tubes. That means the only recourse for pregnancy is IVF. In the case of severe endometriosis, a laparoscopic surgery can be performed to clear away adhesions, which may prevent tubal blockage if the problem is caught before too much damage is done.

Shame, shock, self-blame

When I received my diagnosis, I began thinking back through my sexual history. Confusing sex with love and acceptance, I'd had serial monogamous relationships. Because I had a latex allergy and non-latex condoms were not readily available at the time, I practiced the rhythm method of contraception by abstaining from sex when I thought I was ovulating; simultaneously, my partner used the withdrawal technique.

There were two reasons I didn't seek alternatives or medical advice. First, I thought I was healthy and invincible. Second, I was fearful and ashamed—I didn't want my doctor to know I was sexually active. In fact, I avoided medical doctors for years. For all intents and purposes, I was healthy, happy, and optimistic. I never got sick; I didn't even catch mononucleosis (the kissing disease) when my boyfriend had it. I rarely had medical examinations.

I had conflicting emotions about sex. On the one hand, I thought sex was shameful and wrong, yet on the other hand, I equated sex with love. In the end, I kept silent and barely went to the doctor to do routine checks.

As a result, when I contracted chlamydia but had no symptoms, it went undiagnosed and untreated for decades. This caused pelvic inflammation, which ultimately led to fluid-filled tubes. Only when my fertility doctor found hydrosalpinx did he go back and do a blood test. It revealed antibodies to chlamydia, which meant I'd had a chlamydia infection that was no longer active.

Not happy thoughts

Did my fertility challenges make me less of a woman? Was I a fraud as a TCM practitioner who treated women for fertility challenges? Was I an overall failure in life because of the choices

I'd made? These were honest (albeit momentary) thoughts that crept into my darkest hours.

I don't think I truly believed I was a lesser woman because I couldn't conceive, but the thought passed through my head when I got emotionally charged, just as it had for so many women who'd shared similar thoughts with me in my treatment room. That, in turn, gave me important insight as a practitioner into how normally vibrant, dynamic, otherwise healthy, and still relatively young women could be so thoroughly undermined by a diagnosis of infertility.

It also gave me insight into their inconsolable despair at failing to conceive month after month, no matter what anyone said to encourage and support them. Over the years, I witnessed most of my patients eventually have children, but that didn't alleviate my stress. The fact remained that, no matter how supersonic my husband's sperm were, they would never be able to meet my eggs without considerable help.

Embracing Western medicine

Because my fallopian tubes were blocked, my only chance at conception would be through IVF (the petri dish method). That was not how I'd envisioned making a baby, but that was exactly what we did. Having avoided Western medicine for most of my life, I now embraced it.

I had always been fascinated by science, but never in a million years had I expected to be a human science experiment, especially after watching my grandmother's near-death experience where Western medicine had nothing to offer her. Since becoming a TCM practitioner, my mission had been to have Western medicine embrace and integrate Chinese medicine. I didn't expect that part of my personal growth would be to embrace Western medicine. Although IVF is a well-established procedure, I call it a science experiment because every woman responds differently to the hormonal drugs used to stimulate egg growth. One woman may require very few drugs to coax many egg-containing follicles to develop, while another requires triple the amount of drugs to develop a few follicles. But you don't know how you will respond until you undergo IVF. My own fertility doctor told me after the first failed IVF cycle that it was virtually a test (a very expensive test) to see how I responded to the drugs.

I stepped outside my comfort zone and surrendered, not once but eight times, to IVF. Six of those times progressed to IVF transfer. I discuss the other two times a bit later in this chapter. IVF involves everything from oral medications and injectable hormones to daily blood draws, vaginal ultrasounds, and invasive surgeries. This made eight attempts a stretch for a person who never even took aspirin, and it was demanding physically, emotionally, and, of course, financially.

As noted earlier, the psychological stress associated with infertility is similar to that of a life-threatening illness.[1] Indeed, in my practice I'd watched many women who appeared to be on top of the world suddenly have that world come crashing down on them on learning they faced barriers to conceiving. Many became depressed due to feeling they were out of control when their period arrived. Many isolated themselves from friends and family to avoid talking about such a private issue.

I vowed I wouldn't end up like that and tried to remain hopeful, focusing on those who had become pregnant against all odds. I would allow myself to be sad each time I got my period, but instead of getting sucked into a vortex of despair, I would remind myself to be grateful I wasn't going through menopause.

Reframing my perspective

I must confess that, before all of this happened to me, I considered IVF an act of desperation to be avoided. But walking down the same path forced me to open my eyes and my heart, to reframe my perspective, to see ART more as an opportunity for a second chance than a last resort.

Because my eggs could not meet sperm, I had to evaluate whether I really wanted to have a child through my womb. I knew I did, and I knew it meant IVF. I could either choose it kicking and screaming or I could embrace Western technology and be thankful to have the choice. I chose the latter.

Choosing IVF meant injecting and ingesting hormonal drugs for periods of time. Coming from a holistic background, this made me uncomfortable, so I came at it from a deeper place and one that is more difficult to explain. I can only liken it to a mother risking her life for her child, except in this case I was a potential mother risking the side effects the treatments might have on my body to respond to a profound yearning for my unborn child—a natural, maternal instinct I couldn't deny.

Hurtful things people say to women pursuing IVF

Have people said things like this to you? How does it feel to hear these things? When people in your life say these things, I think they have good intentions, but they lack awareness of how hurtful their words are.

"If you can't have a child naturally, it's not meant to be."

I had someone say this to me directly. She didn't mean to be hurtful, but her words made me feel like a substandard human, not deserving enough to have a baby.

"People shouldn't be treated for medical problems unless their lives depend on it."

First of all, infertility can be a complex medical condition that affects body and mind. What people who say this do not see when they look at people like me is that they are suffering inside. To survive and procreate are basic human instincts that cannot be denied.

"You can just always adopt. Having children is a selfish act, anyway."

My own brother said this to me at one point. I was really surprised and didn't have the energy to let him know how hurtful it was. I was thinking, "Easy for you to say when you have two beautiful daughters. If I want to adopt, let me come to it in my time after I mourn the loss of my potential genetic child."

I'm not sure if having children is a selfish act. Is it selfish for animals to procreate in the wild? It's part of our survival instinct to procreate. Women and couples going through this can't just turn off a switch.

Besides, adoption is not so easy. In fact, we also went through the adoption route in our quest to have a child. I will discuss adoption more in Chapter 9.

Supporting myself on my journey

TCM and acupuncture were of great comfort to me throughout my journey. They helped me manage my stress levels, minimize drug side effects, and increase my ovarian and uterine blood flow. Combining Eastern and Western medicines gave me peace of mind, knowing my husband and I were doing everything we could to optimize our chances of getting pregnant rather than staying stubbornly stuck to one position or the other.

My fertility challenges also gave me an opportunity to practice what I preached by creating balance in my life. I changed my work habits by decreasing my workdays from six to five and also decreasing my daily hours. I de-stressed by walking or jogging twice weekly. I went to yoga class once a week and stretched at home daily. I went to see Shawn Gallagher, a hypnotist whose name countless patients had mentioned and who now works with our clinic. She custom-made recordings for me, which I listened to at bedtime every night.

In preparation for each IVF cycle, when I was taking the stimulation drugs, I used acupuncture to increase blood flow and help the drugs circulate to my ovaries and uterus. (In TCM, we believe inserting acupuncture needles at specific sites along the body increases blood flow to the reproductive organs. Theoretically, needles in these insertion points send a message to the brain, which responds by increasing blood flow and creating a relaxation response, which directs more energy to the reproductive organs.)

I also used acupuncture to decrease the joint stiffness and emotional irritability I experienced from the fertility drugs. Between IVFs, I remained strictly gluten-free, sugar-free, and dairy-free, did a cleanse, and took wheatgrass shots daily to clear out excess hormones.

I frequently came down with a wicked sore throat, cough, and phlegm, and my nose became chaffed from going through so many tissues during my sleepless coughing nights, none of which I'd ever experienced. Before IVF, I'd get sick maybe once every five years for a day and fight it off immediately. But with each IVF cycle, I got sick. I'd use herbs and acupuncture again to prevent colds from progressing

Two weeks of torture

The two-week period from when the eggs were deposited inside me until I could take a pregnancy test was sheer torture, and this is also what I see my patients going through. As much as I would tell myself to relax and not think about it, I couldn't help looking for pregnancy symptoms.

This is futile because fertility doctors routinely prescribe progesterone after ovulation to prepare the uterine lining for the embryo. Because of this, many women experience pregnancy symptoms whether they're pregnant or not. It just makes the rollercoaster ride that much worse.

Several days into one of my waiting periods, on a Monday, I went for an hour-long walk after dropping my mother off at the airport. It was slow and enjoyable, but in the end I had a lingering doubt about whether I should be doing this. I never thought I'd get caught up in this sort of neurotic mind game. I thought I was above all that, but I learned I was just human after all.

It was one more day until the much-anticipated blood test, but I couldn't wait. For the first time, I broke down and bought a pregnancy test. I would have used it right away, but we were hosting my goddaughter Emilie's baptism at our house. If the results had been negative, I would have been upset on "her" day.

I tried to stay outside of myself and focus on Emilie and her brother Etienne for the baptism, but my fears and anxiety were still there in the background. Did I do the right or wrong thing by not taking the prescribed baby aspirin daily? I only started it after the transfer, and even then, I had been barely managing it every other day. This was also the first time after embryo transfer that I saw some smearing of dried dark blood in my panties—what did that mean? Was that implantation bleeding?

These types of things played over and over in my head, inducing continual fear. When I felt some pains in my lower abdomen, I'd start wondering: is that implantation and growth, or is it an embryo detaching? I'd wake up at three in the morning, try to meditate, and finally get up forty-five minutes later to purge the garbage lurking in my head by writing it down. And then I'd worry about the detrimental effects of insufficient sleep. That was why I wanted to do the urine test on the weekend before the scheduled blood test on Monday.

Advice for the two-week wait after IVF (and IUI)

The key to surviving the two-week wait is to get to a place where you have peace of mind without regret, knowing you have created a fertile landscape and now you just have to wait and see if you have a healthy seed to grow. This seems like a good time to dispel a few myths about conception.

MYTH: EMBRYOS CAN SLIP OUT OF THE UTERUS

From the moment after you have your embryo transfer (ET), you fear it will fall out of your womb. Your uterus is a potential space like a deflated balloon, which expands with the growth of your baby when you are pregnant. The uterine lining is sticky like strawberry jam to keep the embryo in place. That means after your embryo transfer, it is safe to do the following:

- Urinate and defecate. It's better to go rather than hold it in after an ET to avoid tensing up your uterus.
- Cough and sneeze. No amount of sneezing or coughing will impede implantation. When I conceived Zoe, I had a month-long cold that had me coughing until my ribs hurt.
- Go back to work within 24 hours. For many, work is a good distraction—unless your job involves heavy lifting or you find it overly stressful.
- Fly. Some couples travel out of country for IVF, such as to the Colorado Center for Reproductive Medicine (CCRM), a world renowned clinic. CCRM recommends forty-eight hours' rest before flying home. On the other hand, if you are a flight attendant who is subjected to jet lag, irregular hours, and bending at the waist over twenty-five times per shift, your work can put you at risk. In this case, I would advise you to stay grounded.

- Relax for the day after ET, but then get up and move around. A 2013 study found that bed rest after ET did not improve IVF success rates, as it decreased blood circulation.[2]
- Engage in light activity. Walking stimulates stress-relieving hormones. That said, you shouldn't engage in vigorous exercise, especially if you are at risk for ovarian hyperstimulation (see Chapter 7).
- Have sexual intercourse. A couple of studies support sex as beneficial for implantation as a result of couple bonding[3] and seminal fluid enhancing implantation.[4] However, the stress of IVF lowers most women's libidos. So if you are in the mood, go for it; if not, don't sweat it.

HOW TO MAKE YOUR UTERUS STICKY TO PROMOTE IMPLANTATION

- Laugh. Laughter releases feel-good hormones (endorphins), which decrease the stress response, relax the uterus, and increase uterine blood flow. A study found laughter after embryo transfer increased pregnancy rates by fifteen percent.[5] So watch funny movies, read funny books or magazines, and be around funny people.
- Be true to your emotions. A lot of women think that you have to think positive in order to get pregnant. Acknowledge your stress; don't stress about being stressed. You cannot force positivity (see Chapter 7 for The three Rs of positive self-talk).
- Acupuncture. Acupuncture has the potential to increase your chances of implantation by more than sixty percent when you do pre- and post-ET treatments.[6] The pre-transfer treatment increases blood flow to the uterus to make it sticky, and the post-transfer treatment helps to relax the uterus for implantation.

DOES SPOTTING MEAN IT'S OVER?

No. Please breathe now. There are several reasons for spotting outside of getting your period or having a miscarriage, including:

- The speculum and catheter used to pass through the cervix may have irritated the uterine lining.
- The progesterone supplements used in conjunction with IVF can cause spotting.
- Implantation spotting can occur when the embryo burrows into the uterine lining and implants (this does not happen to all women).

The things I tried

I tried so many things in my quest to conceive: hypnosis, clairvoyance, fertility counselling, books of all types, friends, isolation, family, acupuncture, acupressure, osteopathy, massage therapy, integrated manual therapy, meditation, colonic irrigation, visualization, spirit baby chanting, fertility yoga, walking, running, no running, bed rest, no bending, no lifting, no sweets, no refined carbs, no dairy.

After trying all that, if we still don't conceive, do we assume we didn't do it well enough? Do we think we didn't believe in the process enough, or we didn't want it badly enough? Is it the doctor's fault? Is the procedure to blame? Is it our age? Do we feel awful for all the things we've done and not done in our lives that could have led to this?

I drove myself crazy with thoughts like, "What is balance? Am I becoming unbalanced when I try too hard to be balanced? Maybe I didn't follow Feng Shui well enough in clearing out the old to help bring in the new. I knew I should've sorted out our clutter and had a garage sale . . ."

My IVF attempts

I attempted IVF a total of eight times. The fertility doctor said the first one didn't count because we had proceeded without surgically removing my fallopian tubes. He theorized that the fluid in my tubes could be toxic and preventing implantation of the embryos in my uterus. I took Chinese herbal medicines, hoping to eliminate the fluid, and after several months, an ultrasound showed the tubes looked clear. So we started IVF drugs, but, to my dismay, the fluids came back. We proceeded with the IVF, but I did not get pregnant.

Because I was forty and not twenty, I decided not to risk another IVF with the fluids in my tubes and consented to a *bilateral salpingectomy,* surgical removal of my fallopian tubes. The clinic cancelled two cycles before egg retrieval because my body was over-suppressed with one set of drugs so that when I took the stimulation drugs (which cost thousands of dollars) no eggs grew. Although the doctor did not count these as IVFs, I did count them because I still suffered the emotional, physical, and financial consequences of taking all those drugs to stimulate my ovaries.

When we finally attempted another IVF cycle, I got pregnant but miscarried. As sad as it was, it reassured me that I was able to get pregnant and fueled my persistence in pursuing IVF. I became like a gambling addict waiting for the next big win. I did say at some point I would stop because in reality even a twenty-year-old has only a one-in-five chance of conceiving naturally each month. I was forty-three by this time, so my chances were much lower.

My triple-pronged approach

From this emerged my triple-pronged approach to becoming a mother: we looked into adoption, IVF with donor eggs, and IVF with my own eggs. Through this process, I learned it was more important to me to be a mom than to be genetically connected to my child. Had I not gone through my fertility challenges, I would never have known that.

During our first two years of trying to conceive, I would never have dreamed that I would consider IVF, donor eggs, or adoption. It wasn't until I faced my fertility challenges head-on that I chose IVF. It wasn't until I walked even farther down this difficult path, with four attempted IVFs behind me, that I opened myself to considering both adoption and donor eggs as viable options.

An advantage to using donor eggs instead of my eggs was that the donor would be taking the fertility drugs instead of me. An advantage to using donor eggs instead of pursuing adoption was that rather than adopting a child from China with no background information, we would pick a donor with a detailed profile, including her GPA, photos, family life, health history, and so on. The one we were considering didn't look anything like me, but she was young, pretty, and smart with great aspirations in life. How could I lose, especially if I got to experience pregnancy and the baby was nourished in my womb? This baby might not have been genetically mine but it would have been biologically mine as I nourished and gave it life. All of a sudden, donor eggs sounded better than adoption.

Jean-Louis was not convinced. Donor eggs would be expensive ($20,000 in Canada at the time) and didn't come with any guarantees. He was right. After all the failed IVF attempts and the miscarriage, it would be a gamble. I wondered when I got to be such a risk-taker? As a little girl, I refused to play poker even for pennies, since I couldn't stand the thought of losing. I had only ever bet on a sure thing, and this was far from it.

The important part for me was that I had finally left my shame and regrets in the past and focused my energy on being in the present and playing the cards I'd been dealt. I surrendered to what was and looked for options rather than being tied to how I had first envisioned getting pregnant—naturally.

Living outside of the baby project

When you are in an IVF cycle, it consumes all your time, energy, and emotions: early mornings for blood work and ultrasounds, daily injections of drugs at home, a day for surgical retrieval of egg-containing follicles, a day for embryo transfer back into your uterus, a two-week wait before your pregnancy test. To keep sane, it's important to do things that make you happy outside of trying to conceive.

I didn't drink alcohol, but when I had a failed IVF, I would do things that I wouldn't do when I was in a cycle. I would go snowboarding. I remember going for dinner at the home of a couple who didn't have kids and singing and dancing to a video game called SingStar through their Play Station. I have a competitive edge and wanted to be at the top of the singing charts, so I had to practice. That took my mind away from thinking about a baby, and it was fun, so that was a strategy for several months.

I didn't want to contemplate the thought of failure, but I saw that, the more I resisted, the more it persisted. So in addition to exploring donor eggs and adoption, I also tried to remember the Taoist perspective that we are all part of a moment in time. Nothing matters and there is nothing to contemplate and no need to think about consequences. I chose to live in the moment and let my thoughts—happy, sad, anxious, worried, hopeful—come and go without self-judgement.

Whatever strategies you can find for taking yourself outside of the intense drama of the baby project are vital, not necessarily to succeed in making a baby but to hang on to your own long-term happiness.

Miracles happen

I recall informing a local RE about a former patient of his who had undergone three rounds of IVF without success and who then went on to conceive a healthy baby boy naturally. His response was, "Yeah, miracles happen." It's as if these cases are dismissed as exceptions, but I have observed too many "miraculous" anomalies over the years to discount them so easily.

After a six-year journey, our miracle happened. I am overjoyed and in love with our daughter, Zoe, who came into our lives during the winter of 2012. This miracle would not have been possible had I not surrendered to the unknown, and I'm forever grateful to medical science and the team of professionals who worked with us.

What would I do if I had a second chance?

- I would not to be ashamed about premarital sex. I would understand that sex is not bad or dirty.
- I would be proactive and get Pap smears and blood work regularly to check for anomalies or STI. That alone would have prevented me from getting blocked tubes in the first place.
- I would learn to say no. I would learn not to confuse sex with love.
- I would educate myself about when to ask for help, and I would learn how and when to accept it.
- I would get therapy. Instead of being in serial monogamous relationships, I would learn to deal with issues rather than run away to find a new partner.
- I would learn to commit. Love is commitment and I had difficulties committing. I didn't learn to commit until I met my husband. I learned to deal with the issues at hand when we faced fertility challenges because they were not something I could run away from.

- I would not take my health and fertility for granted (which brings me back to being proactive to get tested above). Just because my grandmothers both had children at forty-six didn't automatically mean I would, too. I would learn to take better care of me.

Of course, I don't regret the life I've had, for if I hadn't walked this path, I would not have this story to tell, and, more importantly, we would not have the child we were meant to have: Zoe, who is the light of our lives and the love in our hearts.

Why am I sharing my story?

I'm telling my story to empower you to be proactive and educated about your own fertility. The more we're willing to talk about it, the more we're able to diminish the stigma, guilt, and shame associated with fertility challenges.

To take charge of your fertility, get tested early and get treatment for things that can potentially affect your ability to conceive, such as unhealthy weight, sexually transmitted infections (STI), endometriosis, blocked fallopian tubes, polycystic ovaries, thyroid insufficiencies, irregular menstruation, hypertension, or diabetes.

Also, be open to different approaches. Every medicine has its own tool kit. Combining more than one therapy provides many more means to deal with your issues. It's not about giving up what you believe in, whether by trying TCM for the first time when you've never considered an alternative before, or trying Western medicine when you've felt it had nothing to offer you. It's about opening yourself to all the possible ways you can find help on your pathway to pregnancy.

9
Million-Dollar Babies

Breathing in, I calm body and mind.
Breathing out, I smile. Dwelling in the present
moment, I know this is the only moment.
THICH NHAT HANH

Ann: How far would you go?

Ann raced into my clinic after running several blocks from her
office in her business suit and heels. She was thirty-six, a lawyer
who worked in local government. She apologized for being
three minutes late and immediately warned me that she had a
tight schedule and would need to be out on time so she could
get to her next meeting. I told her I'd keep track of time for her,
and, with a laugh, I said she could now hurry up and relax.

She and her husband, Doug, had been trying to conceive
for three and a half years. The first year they tried naturally.
The second year, a fertility clinic diagnosed her as having unexplained infertility (see Chapter 1) but then found that she had
a high follicle stimulating hormone (FSH) and low antral follicle count (AFC), which are both markers of poor ovarian
reserve (POR, see Chapter 3), as well as a thin uterine lining.

High FSH meant that giving Ann FSH in preparation for IVF
would likely not help. Low AFC suggested that fewer eggs

would be available to stimulate for IVF. By clinic standards, a uterine lining (which sheds during menstruation but builds up again in preparation for sustaining an embryo through the first trimester of pregnancy) must be at least eight millimetres thick for implantation and pregnancy to occur.

That said, both FSH and AFC can change from cycle to cycle and are not as accurate as measures of ovarian reserve as fertility specialists once thought they were. Based on these two factors, it might have been more accurate for Ann's RE to say. "This month isn't a good month, as right now you'd likely be a poor responder. We could wait for a month when your FSH is lower and your AFC is higher."

Obsessing about numbers: Just don't

I encourage my patients to avoid obsessing about the numbers from their blood work and the statistics about infertility. I tell them to think of the day they have their blood tests as a moment in time—a snapshot, not a permanent picture. In fact, for any of the conditions that contribute to POR, I have stories about patients who have become pregnant and had babies naturally, despite having the wrong numbers in their bloodwork. For example:

- I've had patients with high FSH get pregnant naturally and have babies, as well as patients who, over the course of TCM treatment, have lowered their FSH levels and become pregnant.
- I've had patients with low AFC become pregnant and carry a healthy baby to term, as well as patients who have increased their AFC over the course of TCM treatment and become pregnant.
- I've had patients whose uterine lining, over the course of TCM treatment, thickened, as well as patients whose uterine lining never hit the eight-millimetre mark and yet have become pregnant and carried a healthy baby to term.

More than half of the women coming to my clinic have elevated FSH, low anti-mullerian hormone (AMH, another marker of POR discussed in Chapter 3), and possibly thin uterine lining, as well. And most of them go on to have healthy babies within two years of starting to work with our clinic. But often doctors get stuck on the dogma about maternal age—that with every passing month, the ovaries and eggs are getting older. They tell a woman she's a poor responder, and she's stuck with that label in her head.

Ann's pre-TCM journey

Ann had already been through quite a lot before the day she ran through my door. In 2004, when she first started her journey with the fertility clinic, she and Doug had tried three IUIs unsuccessfully for three consecutive months. After this, Ann wanted to go straight into IVF before she "ran out of eggs." Her doctor considered her a poor candidate for IVF based on her test results, but that didn't turn out to be the case. She had good quality embryos throughout but produced only two or three of them for each IVF cycle. The doctor recommended they try four IVFs; they did five without a pregnancy.

Ann then connected with an agency specializing in gestational carriers (surrogates). Their surrogate, Tina, had an early miscarriage, but because she did become pregnant, Ann and her husband tried another IVF cycle with Tina the following month.

Women and their fertility doctors are always eager to keep going and launch into another IVF cycle for fear of running out of time. I advise against back-to-back cycles to allow the body to return to balance after being bombarded with drugs. Even though it was Ann's surrogate who miscarried, I would have suggested she allow herself time to mourn this loss. But she was determined and powered on.

By the time Ann came to me, Tina was pregnant. Ann and Doug had now undergone eight IVF cycles, two using a surrogate. Even though they'd already spent $200,000, she didn't want to stop there. Her doctors said she had a "short window of time" before her eggs expired, so she wanted to undergo four IVF retrievals to bank as many embryos as possible to increase their odds of having more babies.

With her baby on the way through her surrogate, Ann decided to make the time to add acupuncture to her medical approach, hoping, as research[1] indicated, that it would be good for her fertility. After just three treatments, Ann's doctor told her doctor that her uterine lining looked good during that morning's intrauterine (or transvaginal) ultrasound. Adding acupuncture was the only change in her regimen.

I thought her uterus was capable of carrying life and she might try an IVF using her own womb again. But in Ann's mind, that ship had sailed, and she was actually relieved she didn't have to carry a baby. So she continued with her plans. The doctors retrieved seven eggs that cycle, three of which fertilized and developed into embryos, which they froze. Then, as soon as she began menstruating, Ann started another IVF stimulation cycle.

During one of our acupuncture sessions in September, Ann told me that Tina had delivered her infant, Haley, who died in the womb after having survived the whole pregnancy. Words could not describe her sense of loss. Nothing had prepared them for a stillbirth. Just when they thought they were finally going to have a family, they were "back at the drawing board" and "starting over from scratch," as Ann said.

At this point, I prescribed Bu Yin Tang, herbs to help calm her spirit, while we continued with acupuncture to decrease her stress response. She had insomnia, was restless, and was experiencing anxiety and depression. This also indicated that her energy and blood flow were going into protective-survival mode, which would, according to TCM principles, reduce the blood flow and energy to her ovaries and uterus just when she needed them to conceive.

Encouraging Ann to take a break

I understood Ann's need to aggressively pursue IVF and try again to become a parent. So many women I work with elect to keep going; their yearning is so strong that they see no other option. For many, doing everything in their power in pursuit of pregnancy becomes a type of therapy. Ann felt the only way to fill the void after Haley's death was to try for another baby. So with more determination than ever, Ann and Doug pursued IVF with a new surrogate.

At the same time, I wanted her to take a break. IVF is physically and emotionally taxing. After she'd done so many rounds of IVF drugs back to back, I felt her body needed to clear out the excess hormones to help her respond better to future cycles. Just as your tolerance for any kind of medicine can increase the amount you need to achieve the same results, a woman may need more IVF drugs to continue producing follicles, or the drugs may stop working altogether because the body stops responding. Also, in Chinese medicine, when you are given drugs to grow follicles, we say that it taxes the body's energy (essence).

My wishes notwithstanding, a month later, Ann started another round of IVF drugs and, after a couple of months, reported feeling depressed. She was not responding well to IVF this time, making fewer, if any, embryos. The doctor now told her she had the AFC of a forty-five-year-old, the lowest she'd ever had. For the next six months, and with each subsequent IVF, the fertility clinic transferred frozen embryos to the surrogate, along with a fresh embryo if Ann had one, but none resulted in pregnancy.

At this point, Ann was in a state of panic. She believed she was one step closer to menopause, even though she was only thirty-six years old, and her poor response to the IVF drugs convinced her this was true. Although I validated her sense of utter devastation, I had my own theory about her failed IVF cycles.

A TCM view of Ann's failed IVF cycles

From my perspective as a TCM practitioner, I did not believe Ann was entering menopause. Instead of basing my opinion solely on statistics and lab numbers, I looked at her overall situation. Ann's physical, energetic, and emotional environment had been disrupted, which can have a profound impact on cellular health. She had been trying to conceive for almost four years at a cost of hundreds of thousands of dollars. She was facing as stressful a health issue as any life-threatening illness, and she'd lost a baby to stillbirth just two months earlier. Not surprisingly, she was depressed.

In my opinion and experience, Ann's poor lab and ultrasound results reflected that, although she desperately wanted a baby, her body went into fight-or-flight mode to protect her, leaving no room or energy to create life. It was her body's way of saying, "No, not now. Let's not force a baby into this world right away. Let's recuperate and harness energy first." But my perspective was very different from that of Ann's fertility doctors, who believed every month that she didn't pursue IVF was wasted.

Despite all the negative results, and my urging that she rest and recuperate, Ann was more determined than ever to have a baby. After another IVF cycle, four embryos were transferred into her surrogate, but she did not become pregnant. Finally, though, Ann noticed her stress increasing with each IVF. Going to the fertility clinic was a constant reminder of her past failed IVFs, negative experiences, and painful losses. She also started to experience whole body aches after her last egg retrieval.

"IVF failed, so I failed"

When a woman has a failed IVF, she tends to take it personally. Instead of saying the IVF failed, most women think, "I failed." This is especially hard for a person like Ann, who always worked hard and got what she was striving for.

Although I disagreed with Ann's choice to keep pushing forward, I was pleased that she was continuing to come to my clinic. Using acupuncture, I did my best to mitigate her mounting stress and increase blood flow to her ovaries to nourish her developing follicles. I also gave her herbs to counteract the side effects of the IVF drugs.

With time, her AFC increased, but the results were still not what she'd hoped for. It was as if she was a fertility gladiator and I was keeping her alive by treating her battle wounds, but they never quite healed because she kept re-entering the arena for another round of fighting. This went on for months. She would cycle in and out of IVFs, sometimes taking a break. I would see her for acupuncture and then she would disappear for several months.

Then one day, Ann came to my clinic with a new plan.

Ann's big bang cycle

Determined to have a baby within a year, Ann wanted to up her game. She lined up five people for an IVF cycle: herself, her sister Grace, an anonymous twenty-something donor whom she'd carefully selected through an egg donor agency, and two gestational surrogates, Petra and Andrea.

The procedure was complex because the fertility doctor had to line up Ann's menstrual cycles with her two egg donors so they would all have matured eggs ready to retrieve around the same time. IVF resulted in embryos from Ann and one of the donors, and the fertility clinic transferred two embryos to each surrogate. Petra and Andrea both became pregnant but

Petra miscarried at eight weeks. Andrea went on carrying twins.

Finally, Ann was optimistic. She went out more and started to enjoy life again. She visited Andrea regularly, taking her out to eat and making sure she was doing well and had everything she needed. At thirty-eight weeks, Andrea delivered two small baby girls, Claire and Rachel, who are now thriving seven-year-olds.

The whole time Andrea was pregnant, Ann kept up with her regular acupuncture treatments. She thought she might want to do IVF again, and she knew acupuncture was helping to decrease her stress levels. She also recognized the need to treat her health imbalances after having taken drugs for three IUI cycles and twenty IVF procedures over five years, with few breaks.

Gradually, Ann's periods returned to normal, with substantial menstrual flow like it had been eight years earlier, before all of the IVF cycles. Emotionally, she was feeling wonderful. She was sleeping through the night (she hired a night nurse to help her feed her babies at night) and happily carrying her two babies around and enjoying her life through her days.

Ann's beyond-belief baby

Several months passed when Ann didn't come to the clinic. I assumed she was busy with her family. As I found out later, her absence was because she thought she was spontaneously going into menopause or, worse, had ovarian cancer.

"It took me nine weeks to realize I was pregnant. The first period I skipped was not a big deal. It wasn't unusual because my body...had been all over the map for eight years. The second period was weird and by then I definitely had some uncomfortable body feelings, but the odds of my having gone into menopause were certainly more likely than what ended up happening. So at nine weeks—because I had to see my doctor and say 'something is off with my body, I'm physically exhausted and I've missed a couple of periods'—I had to take a pregnancy test to basically rule it out. But I was pregnant." After twenty IVFs, no personal pregnancies, a miscarriage and a stillbirth through one surrogate, no pregnancies with a second surrogate, a miscarriage with a third surrogate, and then finally, five years after she started, twins with her fourth surrogate, Ann spontaneously conceived and, at full term, gave birth to a healthy daughter, Emily.

How did Ann get pregnant naturally?

When I interviewed Ann recently for my book and asked her why she thought she became pregnant on her own, she wasn't sure. I asked if she thought it was because she was happy with her twins, allowing her to spontaneously conceive. She did not believe happiness was a factor. She felt she was at her happiest when her first gestational carrier, Tina, was pregnant with her first baby. If the magic bullet was happiness, she believed she should have become pregnant naturally at that time.

I know Ann was happy at that time, but I also know she was working long hours. Although she loved her work, she was far from relaxed. I could see it on her face when she came in for her acupuncture treatments. She would race in to our treatment room looking tense and a little worn out, and after an hour of acupuncture, she would walk out looking more relaxed. They were her "hurry up and relax" sessions, but they were inevitably followed by more meetings and more fires she had to put out. She was used to running on adrenalin, and she thrived on it.

But stress is still stress, even when it's passionate-about-your-work stress; your body does not know the difference between good and bad stress. It's normal to have stress in our lives, but when it over-accumulates, like steam in a pressure cooker, something's gotta give.

Also, at the same time Tina was pregnant, Ann was still undergoing IVF month after month, trying to retrieve as many eggs as possible to create good embryos for a future child. Those procedures added physical stress to her body, which I'm not sure she recognized. In Chinese medicine, we view this as draining her overall life force energy, Qi.

Ann was an intelligent and logical woman who had great survival instincts. She was the kind of woman who would keep running if she twisted her ankle in a marathon just to reach the finish line. She was focused and headstrong. In surviving the fertility clinic, she stayed focused on her goal, the light at the end of her tunnel—a baby. She refused to recognize the accumulation of physical and emotional stresses that had built up over the years of trying to conceive.

I had been treating Ann regularly for much of this time. I saw her through challenges and successes. I know she was happy when Tina was pregnant, but after the birth of her twins, there was an almost palpable difference in her body, mind, and spirit. She was on maternity leave for eight months, so she was no longer experiencing the adrenaline rush of her workday, and she was not being physically or mentally taxed as she had been for years by twenty IVF procedures and disappointments. I am confident that the significant balance she finally achieved created a positive environment for conception.

I recall her coming in for acupuncture just two weeks after her twins Claire and Rachel were born. I was amazed to see how rejuvenated she looked. With the ordeal of her fertility struggles behind her, and without the stress and demands of her crazy work schedule, she was relaxed (or as relaxed as you can be when you are taking care of twins). Because she'd hired a night nurse, she was sleeping through the night. In fact, she was bored at times, missing the intellectual stimulation she was used to.

She was also exuding love, which she was able to express to her twins. This kind of social connectedness contributes to positive emotions that promote better health.[2] Studies have shown that blood pressure drops when someone has romantic love. Stress hormone levels also drop, allowing more blood and energy to redirect itself back to other body parts, such as the reproductive system.[3, 4] I strongly feel these distinct changes in Ann's environment contributed to improved function in her ovaries and uterus, which may have allowed for natural conception. To my mind, this was a clear case where love healed.

The more important question here and how it relates to you is, can you conceive spontaneously when you do not have the financial means (or the physical and emotional stamina) to endure twenty IVFs and use a surrogate or donor eggs to conceive?

The answer is that it is possible. We see this in our practice all the time, as you have seen throughout this book. The paths different women take may vary greatly, but most of them do go on to conceive, some using assisted reproductive technology (ART) and others naturally. Others move on from the fertility fight and opt to adopt, while still others choose to live child-free. I'll talk more about these options in the Conclusion.

Ann's story was far from typical

As I noted at the beginning of this chapter, Ann's pathway to pregnancy was not typical. Her story covers virtually all the different options available through fertility clinics. This journey requires determination, and tests your patience, persistence, and perseverance, but it also teaches something about the healing power of love, whether it's self-love, love of a partner, love of family, or love of friends.

However, Ann's story also illustrates how prohibitively expensive fertility treatments can be. In all my years of practice, I have never seen another couple who have undergone twenty rounds of IVF. She didn't disclose the total costs at the end of their fertility journey, but if they'd spent over $200,000 after eight rounds of IVF and the use of two surrogates—well, you do the math.

The reality for most people

The truth is that the average North American couple cannot afford to pay privately for ART. Cost is the greatest barrier when each IVF cycle, for example, can cost tens of thousands of dollars depending on the clinic, the procedures, and the tests you choose. Pricing typically does not include the drugs required for many of the procedures, and those can add thousands of dollars per cycle. The additional cost of donor eggs, donor sperm, and gestational carriers may add up to far more than the IVF itself.

Even if you never go further than IUI, you're still making a significant investment for each cycle. Another expense is the cost of freezing embryos, which fertility clinics suggest more often since research done in 2015 showed that frozen embryo transfer (FET) may improve pregnancy outcomes by close to nine percent over fresh embryo transfers.[5]

If you live in Canada, different provinces offer limited government subsidies to offset the high cost of IVF treatment, and you may be able to claim your costs as a health expense on your annual taxes. State governments in the US offer no subsidies, although there may be tax breaks for IVF costs and some private health insurance plans cover the cost of drugs and an IVF. My husband was working at a large company, which offered enough funding to cover the fertility drugs we required for one IVF cycle.

More couples are opting to check for chromosomal abnormalities (now very common) by doing pre-implantation genetic screening (PGS). This improves the success rate of IVF, but can cost a significant sum for each batch of embryos. If this had been available when Ann was going through her ordeal, she might have saved time and money by implanting only normal embryos rather than transferring them blindly, where perhaps some of the negative results were due to chromosomal issues. That would have also saved a great deal of emotional turmoil.

Currently, more and more women are doing three rounds of IVF retrieval cycles to bank embryos. At each egg retrieval, the fertility clinic would do a biopsy on one cell from each fertilized egg at the five-to-six-day mark (when the embryos are multi-celled) and then freeze them. Once they have done three rounds of IVF retrievals, they test these biopsied cells all at once. At a later date, they transfer back the chromosomally normal embryo(s) into the woman's womb.

The financial repercussions of fertility treatments can continue years into the future. I've seen people go into debt, or sell or refinance their homes to pay for these treatments, all of which adds to the stress of an already stressful journey. From what I see at my clinic every day, the greater the financial investment, the greater the emotional investment. So when you don't get pregnant, your disappointment and feeling of being out of control increase exponentially.

IVF may increase the possibility of pregnancy, but it's not a magic bullet. A recent UK study recommended doing up to six cycles of IVF to achieve a live birth.[6] That means, from the time you start, you are committing tens of thousands of dollars to cover the costs for at least six IVFs. That puts it out of reach for most people not only financially but emotionally and physically.

Some countries do pay for IVF, including Belgium, the Netherlands, Sweden, Denmark, Finland, and Australia.[7] This social support may lessen the stress levels for citizens of those countries.

Treating complex problems with simple solutions

In Chinese medicine, one of my teachers always says that it is best to treat a complex problem with a simple solution. So instead of throwing everything into the mix, like a whole host of drugs, place a little trust in what you can do with dietary and lifestyle changes. You will feel better, and that alone can help you feel more balanced and connected. From there, you can learn to reduce your stress, cultivate loving relationships, and so on.

The medicalization of baby-making makes us feel inadequate when we can't do such a simple thing—one that is meant to be natural—without help. We live in a world where we believe that doing more will create a better outcome, but baby-making doesn't work that way. Sometimes, the more interventions we use, the more we're likely to feel off centre and off balance. Often what we need to do is be receptive to our bodies' own wisdom (see Chapter 4).

Even if we do decide to follow a medical route, that doesn't mean we have to forget to listen to our bodies. Yes, a doctor's tool box is typically filled with drugs and aggressive interventions. Sometimes, those interventions are warranted. Other times, we could cut back on the interventions and focus on the basics, or at least do both at the same time. In other words, we could bring Eastern and Western medicine together.

No matter what Western medicine says about your AFC, FSH, AMH, or uterine lining, it doesn't mean you can't get pregnant. Some conditions, like mine, preclude pregnancy without assistance, but Ann's story demonstrates that, even after you've tried everything, completely natural miracles can still happen.

Ann's surprising benefits

What Ann says now about acupuncture: "It ended up being an excellent decision. It helped my body overall and I could feel a very real shift take place in how my body was functioning... you were the best health care practitioner I encountered in my fertility journey and you looked at my body in a holistic way, which was different from other practitioners, who looked at their specific role connected to one part of my body."

Why do I share Ann's story? Partly because it's an extreme story of fertility against all odds. But more than that, because as you embark on your fertility journey, you have to ask yourself, even if you don't know the answer yet, when and where you will draw the line. When will you have had enough? How will you know? How open will you be about what you are doing in your effort to have a child? What price will you be willing to pay, not only in dollars but in personal stress, strain on your relationship, and impacts on your body?

Ann's ability to carry on for so long came from her logic and determination. She focused on the here and now, yet had plans for the future. Her logical, practical mind kept her going and minimized her emotional despair.

"Most people don't have the ability to do one [IVF], let alone twenty, and also Doug and I were on the same page, which was a very important factor. Neither one of us wavered, especially because twenty is such an unusual number. It really sounds like we were just throwing money down a rabbit hole.

"But if you lay it out, it's all logical. It was a ton of work to try and fight and build our family, but knowing we could do it successfully once, we felt like we could do it successfully again. That is what kept us going. The total clarity that becoming a parent was something that was very important to me, the desperation in that it had gone on for far too long"—five years and it never stopped.

"There was an element of desperation, and real determination. The only way we were going to become parents was to keep trying...so not trying meant there was a real outcome that wasn't going to happen."

In the end, it did happen, and now as she walks down the street she chuckles.

"People may judge and see me as 'fertile Myrtle.' In reality, they have no idea about the catastrophic journey I had [to go] through to get here."

10

Female-Only Pregnancy

The secret to thriving is the knowledge that we are never
simply victims of our bodies. It's very reassuring to
know that we all have within us the ability to heal from
anything and go on to live joy-filled lives.
CHRISTIANE NORTHRUP, *WOMEN'S BODIES, WOMEN'S WISDOM*

Katherine and Sophie: Two moms

This book wouldn't be complete without a chapter celebrating
the female-only pathway to pregnancy. I want to acknowledge
the particular challenges of women seeking help with conception outside of the heterosexual partnership paradigm. Forty
years ago, trying to conceive in a lesbian relationship or as a
single woman was rare. Today, we see non-traditional family-
building on a daily basis at our clinic.

The following are two stories of hope, with tips to demystify
the challenges you might encounter and help you optimize
your chances of conceiving while minimizing your stress. The
challenge my patients face in both of these stories is lack of
sperm. I hope this chapter will help you choose the options
that are right for you.

Many little girls know from a very young age they want to
have and nurture children. This need goes beyond societal

expectations. A 2007 Finnish study[1] surveyed more than 1500 people, including heterosexual and lesbian women, as well as men. Seventy-eight percent of the women and fifty-eight percent of the men expressed a strong desire to have a child of their own. Women's strong desire could be described as either a "constant longing" that started at a young age, or a "surprising longing" emerging from an unexpected change in perception and experience. The researcher described this biological drive as a "tsunami," meaning a force that could not be controlled.

The study further divided these longings into three groups: women who were triggered by age; women who were triggered by being in a loving relationship and talking with their partners about a future together with children; and women who'd had the "mental and physical experience of being pregnant," meaning they'd experienced miscarriage or had children and had experienced the pregnancy hormones, which triggered the maternal drive. Gloria (Chapter 2) had never considered having children until she was nearly forty; her age, and then her experiences with having a child and miscarriages both triggered her longing for a second child.

If you are a single woman or a woman in a same-sex relationship with the maturity, self-confidence, emotional and financial stability, and supportive community to back you up, nothing is stopping you from conceiving except lack of sperm. Today, science gives you the opportunity to create a family, and TCM can help you create a nurturing, healthy environment into which to welcome and grow a healthy baby.

When reproductively healthy heterosexual couples decide they want to conceive, they rarely seek medical assistance. But in my experience working with same-sex-couples and single women who want to have a child biologically, their lack of access to sperm becomes a fertility challenge requiring assistance, which they can often only get from a fertility clinic.

Despite the fact that lack of sperm is their only impediment to conception, many of my same-sex or single female patients tell me the fertility clinic required them to go through all the same testing as heterosexual couples who arrive at the clinic after having tried to conceive unsuccessfully for a year. Many of my patients say they felt like the fertility clinic was looking for something wrong with them, causing them undue stress.

At the TCM clinic, same-sex couples comprise ten percent of our patient population, and single women comprise another five percent. Our local fertility clinic tells me approximately twenty-five percent of their patients are same-sex couples, another twenty-five percent are single women, and the balance comprises heterosexual couples.

Gay male couples build families, too. And while I see lots of gay men in our practice, none have come in seeking help making a baby. Because of this, I haven't included them in this chapter. That said, I'd suggest gay men (or any men) take the supplements listed in Chapter 5 to support fertility, and pursue acupuncture and TCM to optimize their little swimmers for procreative purposes.

A lesbian pathway to pregnancy

Katherine was thirty-five years old and had been in a relationship with Sophie for five years when they decided to build a family. Katherine had been diagnosed with endometriosis when she was thirty-two and that, combined with her age, made her question her ability to get pregnant. But she worried less about her age when her sister became pregnant naturally at forty.

Before coming to my clinic, Katherine and Sophie consulted a fertility clinic for testing. The first doctor was awkward with them, which made them uncomfortable. He was even more off-putting when he suggested Sophie should conceive rather than Katherine because Sophie was three years younger and didn't have endometriosis. Katherine told me she came away from that appointment feeling a little shameful. The second doctor they consulted was more encouraging, telling them lots of women have endometriosis and get pregnant. Katherine and Sophie opted for non-medicated IUI using sperm from an unknown donor with an open ID.

On her own, Katherine changed her eating habits, consuming more organic foods and eliminating packaged foods, junk food, refined sugar, carbohydrates, and coffee. She started taking prenatal vitamins, and one month prior to trying to conceive, she went from having ten cigarettes per day for twenty years to none.

The missing link: Donor sperm

The pathway to pregnancy for a lesbian couple or a single woman requires sperm, which can be a considerable challenge when there is no guy in the picture. This requires a sperm donor, which may also be the case for heterosexual couples when the male partner lacks sperm (see Chapter 5). Finding a sperm donor can be a complex and stressful endeavour. As with most aspects of building a family, there is no one right way to do this, but there is a way that's right for you.

There are three options to consider when using donated sperm: the known donor, the unknown and anonymous donor, and the unknown donor with open ID.

KNOWN SPERM DONOR

The known donor may be someone who is already in your life, like a brother or a friend. It may also be someone you don't know initially but get to know in order to make a connection and an arrangement.

PROS:

- You know the donor and all his physical attributes as well as his mental, emotional, and physical health and his family history.
- If you want him in your child's life and that is prearranged explicitly in a legal contract, your child can have an open relationship with him.
- You do not have to pay for the sperm, although you may pay for IUI, unless you do self-insemination at home.
- You'll have more information to offer your child about the father, even if he is not in your child's life, so he or she can avoid the pain of fabricating or fantasizing about their unknown father.
- If and when your child needs information about his or her genetic inheritance, such as for medical purposes, that will be readily available.
- In an extreme medical emergency, you will have access to the donor's blood relatives, who could, for example, be screened as organ donors.
- The experience will be more personal for all participants.

CONS:

- Federal agencies in Canada and the United States require that the sperm be tested and quarantined for six months to prevent communication of sexually transmitted infections, which delays the process.
- If the donor is in your child's life, and even if you spell this out in a legal contract beforehand, you may have disagreements about parenting.
- The donor may be able to sue for custody or visitation rights.
- Parenting or custody disagreements can strain dynamics in your immediate and extended families if you have an unanticipated falling out with the donor in the future.

- Although you do not have to pay for his sperm, you might have to travel to acquire his sperm if he lives far away or pay for his travel to you for inseminations.
- After choosing your known donor, you may be disappointed if his sperm analysis indicates STI or poor sperm parameters.

UNKNOWN SPERM DONOR

Sperm banks all over the world offer unknown donor sperm. There are two categories of sperm donors: those who are completely anonymous (the child can never identify him) and those who consent to an identity release option (upon turning eighteen, the child can gain access to information about his or her biological father, but the donor has no legal rights or obligations to the child).

PROS:
- The sperm are carefully screened for diseases and stored at sperm banks.
- Having been tested, the sperm can be used immediately upon selection.
- Donors provide medical, health, and genetic information.
- Donors sign legal documentation waiving parental rights.

CONS:
- Your selection options are limited to the pool of potential donors available at that time.
- The donor is not required to update medical information as time goes on.
- You cannot meet the donor to assess his personality traits; you're limited to the physical descriptions and baby pictures he provides.
- Cost can be prohibitive, as there is a cost per vial of sperm and it can require up to six cycles to conceive for women

between thirty and forty years old (as suggested by a German research article in 2013[2]).

- Your child will have less background information about their genetic father growing up.[3]
- In a severe medical emergency, you and your child do not have access to the donor's blood relatives, who could, for example, be screened as organ donors.
- Your child may have an unknown number of half siblings depending on who else chooses the same donor sperm, or if the donor has children with a partner. This can be stressful for the child.[4]

Because there are so many sperm donor agencies available, it can be stressful trying to decide which sperm bank to choose from before you even begin to look at the donor profiles themselves.

Moreover, there are pros and cons to choosing a completely anonymous sperm donor and choosing a donor with an open ID. For example, anonymous sperm donation ensures complete privacy, which may be valued by heterosexual couples who do not want the child to know they used donor sperm. However, current research supports openness with the child for the same reasons it supports being open with children who are adopted; even if they don't have access to their biological parent(s), openness circumvents numerous psychological issues. However, depending on the sperm bank, you may receive (for extra fees) notes written from donor to potential recipient, or audio interviews, which can provide a sense of connectedness that may be missing for and damaging to the child when the donor is completely anonymous.[5]

The issues involved with sperm donation are many, thorny, and often surprising, so I strongly advise you first, choose a certified and accredited sperm bank, and second, consult a fertility counsellor as well as a legal advisor who specializes in fertility issues and specifically sperm donation. They will have you contemplate scenarios, virtually all of which have arisen in the real world but that you might never otherwise consider, and this knowledge will better guide you to the decision that's right for you.

Trusting your gut

After examining the pros and cons in a rational and thoughtful way, and after consulting a fertility counsellor and lawyer, you may still have difficulty deciding which way to go. I've worked with so many women who had the same trouble coming to a decision about their sperm donor, but when I encouraged them to listen to their instincts, their decisions became clearer.

In Western culture, we are not taught how to trust our instincts but to focus our decision making through our rational minds. However, when it comes to giving birth, which is very much an instinctive impulse, we need to give our inner knowing as much of a voice as our logical minds.

But if you're stressed and worried about making the right decision—or worse, if you're worried you'll make the wrong decision—no decision will get made. And when you're closed off by stress, you're also closed off from receiving important internal signals. Making decisions by relying on only your brain does not necessarily serve your instinctive needs. When you trust your gut, it does not get clouded by excessive thought, worries, and fears.

It is impossible to connect with and get trustworthy information from your gut if you are in a state of panic. Good decisions come from a state of calm and clarity. Most of the fertility decisions you will make require your innate wisdom and ability to be open. You've already examined all of the pros and cons with your logical mind. Now is the time to allow for inspiration.

An experiment in self-trust

Try this experiment. Sit quietly with the lists of pros and cons from the known and unknown donor scenarios. Read one statement, close your eyes, visualize it, and notice how you feel about it. Do you feel uneasy, neutral, or good in your body? That is your gut instinct at work. Make a note of how it feels as you think about each statement. It may help for you to read each statement out loud, which can sometimes foster a sense of clarity.

Listening to your gut requires first clearing your mind. Some may sit quietly and meditate on it. Others may need to physically get the stress out of their bodies by going for a walk or a jog and connecting with nature. Acupuncture, massage, other body work, and hypnosis are other ways to create this calm and connect with your inner voice, which has its own innate wisdom.

Practice slowing down and thinking of the consequences of each choice, and, more importantly, notice how your body reacts to these thoughts. Remember, there is no one right decision. Just do what feels good in your gut and you won't go wrong.

Katherine and Sophie's donor

Like many lesbian couples, Katherine and Sophie first considered a family member, Sophie's brother, to be their sperm donor. They liked the idea that the baby would be tied to both of them genetically. But Katherine felt uneasy about having a known third party who could potentially change his mind and want to parent the child.

Instead, they opted for donor sperm. They made a date night out of it and chose the donor over a glass of wine. Or rather, they made four date nights out of it, sitting by the computer and figuring out who they agreed on. They approached it like an online dating process where they reviewed potential donor profiles from Canadian and American donors. There were fewer donors to choose from in Canada, and their profiles only included photos of eye shapes, nose, and mouths, whereas the ones from the US were full headshots.

Finally, they chose an American donor with open ID so their child would have the option of connecting with him at eighteen. Their donor had features similar to Sophie's. At thirty years old, he was mature, musically inclined, and had a high IQ. They were particularly impressed with the articulate letter he had written to possible donor recipients. They also found out he did not have any live births to date.

After picking their donor, they bought four vials of frozen, pre-washed sperm (that is, the more normal and denser sperm were separated out using a centrifuge, omitting the lighter non-viable sperm and semen). This was done through their fertility clinic, which guaranteed more than 15 million sperm per vial. They used three of the vials before they got pregnant. Single women who want to have a child go through the same process.

Getting started

When Katherine didn't conceive after the first non-medicated cycle of IUI, she smoked several cigarettes and had a few glasses of wine (over a few days) before refocusing and coming to my clinic for acupuncture, counselling, and other pre-conception advice in preparation for another round of IUI.

In addition to the dietary and supplement regime I suggest to my pre-conception patients (see Chapter 1), I prescribed specific Chinese herbs to nourish her constitution, as well as DHA/EPA (fish oils), Wobenzym (women with endometriosis should take this four or five times daily forty-five minutes before food and two hours after food for this systemic enzyme to help break up fibrin scar tissues, and decrease inflammation, swelling, and pain.[6] It can also be used as an immune therapy to prevent miscarriages,[7] along with Royal Jelly, discussed in Chapter 2).

IUI: The simplest ART but still not perfect

When Katherine didn't get pregnant the second time, she began obsessing about it and was constantly online, looking for the next thing to try. At her next acupuncture appointment, I sensed her anxiety and reassured her that she was on the right path, doing everything she could do to optimize her chances to conceive. It was healthy for her to hear that, especially after sifting through heaps of conflicting information.

Although IUI can increase one's chances of conceiving (as the clinic gets the best sperm by spinning it through a centrifuge and inserting it where it needs to go), it's not a guarantee. Not every egg is the right one. In any given cycle, the chance of conceiving is lower than that of not conceiving, which is why even a heterosexual couple needs to have had regular intercourse for a year without pregnancy before fertility is considered an issue.

I explained to Katherine and Sophie that doing an IUI cycle costs time, effort, emotion, and money, which naturally increases stress levels, as do expectations and disappointment when the pregnancy test is negative. According to TCM principles, stress takes energy away from the reproductive organs and can make it more difficult to conceive. I suggested to Katherine that nothing was wrong; she just needed to manage her stress and focus on positive outcomes.

The pot of gold at the end of Katherine's rainbow

Katherine decided to take a break from trying to conceive and instead focused on changing her environment, thoughts, and feelings, continuing with acupuncture and healthy eating practices. She also dealt with a few stresses in her life and, as a result, felt that she knew instinctively when the time would be right to embrace another cycle of IUI. This time, the procedure was successful and we continued treating her for pregnancy support through the first trimester.

As she neared her due date, Katherine was concerned that she would have to be induced if she stayed pregnant beyond her due date at forty weeks. Remembering a conversation we had in her first trimester, she opted to try acupuncture to help prepare for and expedite labour and delivery through a protocol where a woman comes in for acupuncture weekly starting at thirty-six or thirty-seven weeks to slowly help ripen the cervix. When she came in at thirty-seven weeks, we did acupuncture treatments intended to help ripen her cervix, invite labour, and prevent medical induction (which she dreaded). She came in weekly three times and ended up having a smooth and easy labour, giving birth naturally to baby Levi just two days before her scheduled induction date.

Carolyn: A single mom's pathway to pregnancy

More and more women are deliberately setting out to have and raise a child on their own. Typically, these women are highly educated, financially stable, and supported, and I have helped many single women conceive children and start their own families. I will share Carolyn's story with you because it highlights her contemplative journey and the options she considered on her three-year pathway to becoming a single mother. Once Carolyn had decided to move forward with conceiving through IUI and donor sperm, she came to my clinic and started pre-conception treatment.

My pre-conception treatment for women who are planning to have a child on their own is unique in that I counsel women to create a caring community of support at the same time they are undergoing TCM pre-conception treatments, preparing their bodies, minds, and spirits to receive an embryo. With TCM treatments, they are creating and nurturing a healthy physical and emotional environment. By creating a caring community of support, they are endeavouring to bring a baby into a nurturing and loving environment.

At the age of thirty-nine, Carolyn was single and began to consider having a child on her own. She consulted a fertility specialist who presented her with options about procedures she could undergo and information about using sperm donors. She weighed the option of having her eggs frozen but at that time the fertility specialist said the technology hadn't been perfected. She considered having her eggs fertilized with donor sperm and frozen as embryos, which are multi-celled, much larger than eggs, and more stable to freeze. That didn't feel like the right option because she didn't want to eliminate the possibility of having a child with a future partner if she became involved in a long-term, loving relationship.

At that time, however, she realized that she had a deep fear of being a single mom and wasn't confident she could do it on her own. She decided she wanted to be in a loving relationship before embarking on motherhood. Three years later, she was financially stable, had a great life, and was travelling the world. While on a holiday, feeling peaceful and content, she contemplated where her next trip or adventure might take her and was overcome by a strong, undeniable sensation. Suddenly, having a child on her own felt like the best idea she'd ever had.

Carolyn spent the next several hours researching her next steps, and when she arrived home, she started pre-conception treatment with me and began her research about single women in preparation for creating a healthy environment for her child. She was confident that, with positive support around her, she could minimize negative psychological and emotional consequences for her future child. Unlike three years earlier, she felt confident she could do it on her own. Although her heart was set on having a child biologically, she also considered adoption if she was not able to get pregnant.

Creating a community

Creating a community of support is especially important when you are embarking on having a child or children on your own. Having a plan in place and a support system of caring and loving people around you is crucial to ensuring that the environment you want to bring your baby into is full of nurturing energies. I assign my single patients these tasks as homework while they're undergoing pre-conception treatment with me.

BEFORE CONCEPTION

1. I suggest my patients choose specific friends, family, and coworkers to share their news with. Carolyn did this and the outpouring of love and support fortified her confidence in her decision.

2. After identifying your supportive group, invite someone to attend appointments to fertility clinics. Carolyn's sister went with her to all of her appointments.

3. Choose a fertility specialist who is supportive of you and your desire to be a single mom.

4. Keep the statistics in perspective. Carolyn's first meeting with a fertility specialist was full of statistics, like that at forty-two she was reproductively old and her chance of conceiving was five percent. Carolyn gave his remarks a positive spin, saying she would be one of the five percent who have a healthy baby.

5. I remind my patients who are conceiving as single women that they're going to the fertility clinic for sperm. Doctors

may focus on finding a problem because fifty percent of their patients have fertility challenges. As a single woman who's using TCM to enhance your healthy environment, your only challenge is a lack of sperm.

6. I suggest to my single patients to consider inviting trusted friends or family to help choose the sperm donor. It's an important decision, and it should be a calm and joyful experience. One of my patients invited her closest friends to a sperm donor party and she shared with them her short list of possible candidates. Each friend chose their top two candidates. She was thrilled when her five friends each chose the same donor!

PREPARE YOUR BODY

As part of her pre-conception treatment, Carolyn had fifteen acupuncture treatments where I focused on increasing the blood flow to her reproductive organs.

AT IUI OR EMBRYO TRANSFER

1. If you are doing IVF, ensure that you have a trusted friend or loved one with you and to take you home and take care of you. IVF retrieval is a surgical procedure and depending on where you have it done, you will have either sedation or general anaesthesia.

2. Whether for IVF or IUI, I recommend having a family member or trusted friend present to share in the moment when you're being inseminated or doing an embryo transfer. Even though you're in a sterile environment, surround yourself with love and positive energy. Carolyn's sister was with her, holding her hand. When I did my embryo transfers in the surgical room, feet in stirrups, and doctor, nurse, and technician staring at my bottom, my husband would stand by my side and hold my hand. It made the experience a little

nicer for me, and I believe for my baby, Zoe. It's a far cry from romantic sex, but you do what you gotta do.

3. After your procedure, have someone take you home, and make sure your home is a nurturing environment. Have a nourishing meal with your support person, relax, watch a funny movie, and ponder your life with your potential child. One patient asked her father to drive her home from her egg retrieval and his love and support was so comforting that she asked him to be with her and hold her hand during her embryo transfer. What an amazing way for him to be there for his daughter and grandchild.

Baby Jane and Carolyn's village of support

Carolyn had strong support while trying to conceive. So when the first IUI was unsuccessful, she was not alone. Her team consoled her and encouraged her to try again. Her second cycle was successful and she became pregnant with baby Jane. When she was confident her pregnancy was healthy, she expanded her community of support and joined a group of women who were single moms by choice. There she met like-minded women facing similar challenges at different stages of their own journeys. Most of the women were going to sperm banks. Some women had a wider view and were thinking about adoption or foster parenting. The group facilitator as well as the group members were supportive and provided practical advice and information to one another pertaining to their specific circumstances. And since joining, Carolyn has made some lifelong friends.

Carolyn's journey had challenges. She still grieved not having a partner to be with her throughout her pregnancy and in raising her child. She was so pleased that she had pre-arranged support throughout her journey and was grateful that she attended her appointments with her sister, as it was occasionally difficult to see happy couples in the waiting room. But for the most part, Carolyn was very happy throughout her pregnancy, and she appreciated my advice to create her village of support. She said it was a tremendous experience and one of the best periods of her life. But had she not gotten pregnant, she would have been willing to look into adoption.

Adoption challenges and logistics
Although this book is named *Pathways to Pregnancy,* it's also about pathways to welcoming a child into your life. While most of my patients become pregnant, some recognize their stress levels are so high that they need to stop. Although adoption is a stressful process in itself, many patients tell me that focusing their attention on adoption helped to calm their monthly concerns about having a child biologically. While adoption may not be the first choice, many adoptive parents, far from considering adoption an afterthought, last resort, or consolation prize, are deeply grateful for the journey that brought them to the children they love and adore as much as any biological parent ever did.

Things to consider about adoption
Many women who've had fertility challenges heard from some well-meaning friend or relative, "If you can't have kids yourself, you can always adopt." Typically, people make this offhand suggestion with no idea of the complexities associated with adoption. Adoption is a viable way to build a family, but it's not as easy as some might think. For many, adoption is not their first choice, and it takes time to come around to the idea of it; for some families, it never becomes the right choice.

When my husband and I were going through fertility treatments and wanting to stop the emotional rollercoaster ride after multiple failed IVFs, we pursued adoption. Our exploration opened our eyes to the reality that adoption comes with its own set of challenges. For example:

- Depending on the jurisdiction you live in, or the country you wish to adopt from, different rules define your eligibility to adopt. Essentially, you have to meet criteria regarding age, sexual orientation, marital status, physical and mental health, and financial stability.
- In Canada, in more than twenty states in America, and in another twenty countries around the world, you need to complete the PRIDE program (Parent Resources for Information, Development, and Education) as a prerequisite to adopting. This program educates potential foster and adoptive families on how to deal with attachment issues, how best to meet a child's needs, how to help children feel safe and nurtured, and how to help adopted children overcome developmental delays, trauma, and loss.
- In any country, there are costs attached to private or international adoption. In Canada, it is free if you do it through a publicly funded agency, like the Children's Aid Society in Ontario or the Ministry for Children and Families in British Columbia. In the US, the adoption route is free only when you foster to adopt. However, going this route provides no guarantees that you will have permanent placement of the child in care, as the government's goal is always to reunite the birth child with the birth parent.
- Every jurisdiction has different requirements, but virtually all require a home study to be completed by an adoption practitioner, typically a social worker who evaluates your suitability for adoption. This process usually takes from three months to a year to complete.
- The challenges you may encounter vary depending on where you adopt from. For example, many Russian adoption

agencies have babies with fetal alcohol syndrome, while Chinese orphanages are filled with baby girls who were abandoned due to the country's one-child policy.

- There is a possibility that a child who has come through an orphanage will have growth and developmental delays. (For every three months spent in an institution, they may be one month delayed.[8])

I will not deny that we had natural fears around adopting a child with unknown genetics, developmental delays caused by fetal alcohol syndrome, or attachment issues caused by institutional neglect. Despite that, it was encouraging to see studies showing that love, time, and energy (all of which may be lacking in short-staffed orphanages where babies cannot get the one-on-one attention they need to thrive) helps with these challenges, and many babies "catch up" in no time.

Some barriers to adoption

The two most significant barriers to adoption are cost and time:

- There are several costs involved with both private and international adoption. You pay the cost of the home study as well as the costs for documents you need to obtain. In Canada and some other countries, these fees are waived for public adoptions locally. There is a fee for international adoption agencies, which covers staff salaries, operating costs, and legal fees. Depending on the country, these fees can be tens of thousands of dollars. If you are adopting internationally, you will also have travel costs.
- Wait times for adoption can range from a year to many years, and you have no control over this part. For us, after we completed PRIDE and the home study and were subsequently approved by the Canadian agency for eligibility to

adopt through China, we were put on a wait list. Other people on that list had been sitting in the queue for three years and were still waiting. Determined to have a child one way or another and being placed on a wait list with no end in sight pushed us to try IVF again.

At the end of the day, if you have the primal urge to be pregnant and procreate, adoption may not serve that. But do not rule it out either. I have seen plenty of women and couples who start out with a certain set of limitations as to what they are willing or not willing to do to have a child. Through the passage of time and self-reflection, they open their minds to different possibilities, ranging from use of assisted reproductive technologies (ART), to alternative medicines like TCM and acupuncture, or adoption.

The egg-freezing option

When you are a single woman in your thirties, there is a lot to think about: Do you want to try to conceive on your own, or do you wait for the man of your dreams? If the latter, do you consider egg freezing as a way to preserve your fertility? It's a viable and miraculous option if you have cancer and need to undergo chemo and radiation, where the drugs used can shut down your reproductive organs.

However, if you are interested in opting to do this electively as a healthy single woman, you need to know the details. It's not as simple as walking into your nearest fertility clinic to have your eggs sucked out on demand and popped in the freezer. Rather, egg freezing is an art and a science, requiring a complex orchestration that necessitates the use of injectable hormonal drugs and surgery.

Not everyone qualifies. Research indicates that the younger you are (under thirty-four), the better your chances for cryopreservation of your eggs.[9] In order for a fertility clinic to do this for you in good conscience, they would look at your anti-mullerian hormone (AMH) and follicle stimulating hormone (FSH) to see if this pathway is viable for you. These numbers can predict the way you would respond to fertility drugs to maximize egg development.

It is important for fertility clinics to be very deliberate in choosing appropriate candidates for egg freezing. A study from 2013 shows that if you are between the ages of thirty and thirty-nine, you need to freeze an average of twenty-one eggs to create one take-home baby.[10] Typically, the younger you are, the more eggs you have available at any given menstrual cycle to hormonally supersize with injectable drugs and retrieve at ovulation for freezing. It's important to maximize the number of eggs because not all of them will survive the process when you freeze, thaw, and fertilize them at a later date.

It can be a rigorous journey, as it is both physically and emotionally demanding. And from the numbers above, it might also be financially out of reach because each cycle of egg retrieval is expensive, not including drug costs. If you retrieve ten eggs in one cycle, statistically speaking, you would want to do a second cycle to maximize the number of eggs and increase your chances of taking home a baby in the future.

And for each cycle, you need to take oral contraceptives for some time, then egg-stimulation hormones, followed by a trigger shot to ripen your eggs to help their surgical retrieval. Many women experience side effects, including irritability, moodiness, bloating, and headaches, among other things. At the end of the day, the process is gruelling and is not for every woman. But if you feel this is the route for you, TCM and acupuncture can help you maximize your chances for a successful egg-freezing procedure.

Maximizing your egg-freezing prospects

Pre-conception treatment for three to four months prior to egg freezing can maximize your treatment for a successful outcome in the future. We've already learned that *folliculogenesis* (the development of an egg from a resting germ cell to an ovulating follicle) takes 120 days. That means before you embark on egg freezing, you should take time to cultivate your soil (your reproductive organs and specifically your ovaries) to maximize the number of eggs you have available for your harvest. That requires three months.

If you have already gone to a fertility clinic and your blood tests show your FSH and AMH at sub-optimal levels, you might panic and think you are going to run out of eggs tomorrow and be inclined to go straight into an IVF cycle to retrieve your eggs. Instead, take a deep breath and remember from other chapters that these numbers give you a baseline, and there is a possibility they can change for the better by using TCM pre-conception treatments and tips to optimize your ovaries. I see positive results every day.

Three months allows you ample time and opportunity to create harmony and reclaim your natural fertility. Cleanse your body of toxins; eat whole organic, antibiotic-free and hormone-free foods; take appropriate supplements (see Chapter 4); minimize exposure to toxins; and decrease your stress as much as possible. Find a trusted TCM practitioner and have acupuncture treatments to maximize blood flow to your ovaries and induce the relaxation response, which helps optimize reproductive function.

Acupuncture combined with Chinese herbal medicine will help your body find the balance it needs to allow your reproductive organs to function optimally, regulating your periods and treating pre-existing conditions such as endometriosis, polycystic ovarian syndrome, diabetes, thyroid issues, and so on. You may want to try yoga, meditation, or any other types of exercise that encourage a calming effect for you. One of the reasons I suggested in the Introduction that you read the whole book is that you can find tips and advice that focus on pre-conception treatment throughout the book.

Whether you are using donor sperm or freezing your eggs, TCM pre-conception treatments are invaluable in creating a healthy balance while optimizing and preserving your fertility.

If you are a same-sex couple or a single woman, you may be sperm challenged, and, on top of that, you may have other fertility concerns, such as endometriosis or advanced maternal age. But if the circumstances are right, you can follow your pathway to fertility and build a family of your own. And TCM can help you achieve the pre-conception health that will unlock the fertility in you.

11

New Developments and Final Thoughts

Technology is constantly evolving. Every day we are seeing new and controversial contributions to the world of ART. Take for example Augment treatment developed by OvaScience. It evolved based on the research finding egg precursor (stem) cells in the wall of the ovaries, dispelling the belief that women are born with all the eggs they will ever have.

Recently, one of my patients, who was one of a first handful of patients who conceived through Augment, simultaneously did acupuncture throughout her journey. She had her mitochondria (the energy or fuel) of her ovarian stem cells surgically extracted and then injected into the retrieved eggs from IVF to improve egg health, energy, and quality. She gave birth to baby Daniel in April of 2016. The point is, even with the technology, we worked together. (Augment is currently not available in the US, even though the technology was developed there.)

There are several new developments like this on the horizon. Will they make Chinese medicine, acupuncture, and supplements obsolete? That's very unlikely. Augment, for example, works on the principle of extending the energy in a woman's eggs for a longer time, which TCM strives to do by redirecting a woman's energy to her follicles or eggs so they will come to fruition naturally—and it does so at a much lower cost.

In fact, TCM, which aims to improve the ovarian environment with increased blood flow carrying oxygen, energy, and nutrients to help cellular growth, is in line with a new study about how we can intervene with embryo potential.[1] The truth is that, no matter how science progresses in the field of fertility, there will always be room for TCM to help optimize our natural healing power. As Dr. Bruce Lipton puts it, "Western medicine works on the mechanisms and parts of the car whereas Chinese medicine works on the person who drives the car."

Changing the face of family-building

In other words, no matter how complex or daunting your diagnosis or how involved your intervention or treatment, it is crucial to get your body back to balance. Improving pre-conception health and ameliorating physical, emotional, and spiritual well-being will always play an important role in conception.

At the end of the day, life chooses life. The more you are aligned and balanced, the more receptive your body will become to conception, with or without treatment at a fertility clinic. Technology alone will never provide all the answers to every person seeking reproductive help. Helping more people build families requires recognizing and addressing numerous fundamental issues.

However, doing so must begin with recognizing that the drive to procreate is one of the most powerful instinctive drives human beings face. No matter how many women and men put it off in favour of career development through their twenties and thirties, it catches up with most of us eventually. Large progressive corporations have begun to understand this and create supportive family policies. As PowerToFly president Katherine Zaleski said in a 2015 issue of *Fortune* magazine, "Over 80% of us will become mothers by the age of 44, according to the US Census Bureau. So embrace your future and support it at work!"[2]

That said, corporations and governments need to recognize that being family friendly means more than being receptive to women who spend ten or twenty years building their professional lives and then take a few months' maternity leave. There is also a need to recognize that, as long as people continue delaying family-building until their careers are established, one in six employees in any workplace—male or female, heterosexual or homosexual, singles or couples—will struggle with fertility challenges. And those parents-to-be, whether they are going to build their families naturally or through IUI, IVF, surrogacy, or adoption, deserve support, too.

There are signs that this is beginning to happen. As noted in Chapter 6, some workplaces, like Krista's, support women facing fertility challenges, but there remains a huge stigma around admitting such things to family and friends, never mind in the workplace, and there are far too many workplaces like Samantha's, which simply alienate and drive away good employees. We need public education to show employers that building employee loyalty by supporting them through health challenges, including fertility challenges, makes good economic sense in the long term.

"Happier people make more productivity," Larry Page, co-founder and CEO at Google, has said.[3] In 2016, Google was rated the number one workplace in the US by *Fortune* magazine (in seven out of ten years). This was based largely on extensive employee surveys noting employee satisfaction, management styles, pay, and benefits, among other things. In 2015, *Fortune* rated Larry Page the number two CEO in the US. Page's goal, he said, is to make Google a "family" environment, to create happy employees by offering lifestyle perks that support family time, a perk they accommodate by focusing on employees' output instead of on hours worked.

It's progressive thinking, but addressing the needs of those with fertility challenges means going a large step further and thinking about how to support families long before the babies arrive. On the face of it, Facebook and Apple are leading the way. In 2014, these tech giants introduced policies paying up to $20,000 for female employees to freeze their eggs. Clearly, they recognize that encouraging young women to focus on their careers in their twenties has been very good in many industries and good for the economy overall.

Kudos to companies that are beginning to think this way, but they're still way behind the curve. To a woman in her twenties without a blip of marriage or kids on her radar, egg freezing might sound good and logical, but it creates a false sense of security. Frozen eggs do not guarantee a pregnancy. Although a new process called *vitrification* allows for flash-freezing of eggs to prevent crystallization (which is like freezer burn), freezing embryos (fertilized eggs) is still far superior. Not only are embryos larger and more stable to freeze and thaw, but they are three times more likely to create a healthy baby than unfertilized eggs (see Chapter 10).

So offering young women opportunities to freeze their eggs in their twenties and early thirties to hedge their bets in case the right guy doesn't come along or fertility issues arise when they later try to conceive may sound proactive. But it doesn't begin to deal with the heartbreaking stress and exorbitant expense of dealing with fertility challenges, which more often than not remain undiscovered and untreated until women and men try to conceive in their thirties and sometimes forties.

If family policies and egg-freezing policies are not the answers, what are? We can't go back to a time when women stayed at home and had babies in their late teens and early twenties, and nor should we want to. The rapid entry of women into the workforce has been and will continue to be good for both the economy and overall social welfare in any country that's embraced it. If going back isn't the answer, going forward must be—but how?

To me, there are several ways to move forward, but all of them start with recognizing that fertility challenges should not just be dealt with privately in secrecy and shame. They should be discussed publicly and openly, and recognized as a public health issue and a workplace issue that affects one-sixth of the population, and men and women equally. To me, this means:

- There must be public education to reduce the stigma that surrounds fertility issues and discourages people from talking about it and seeking support.
- This education must encourage people to have their fertility health checked as routinely as they would have their blood pressure checked, with an eye to diagnosing problems early and treating them before they get out of control.
- This education must also include recognizing that prevention is the best way to deal with many health issues, including fertility issues. While Western medicine is good at responding to health issues after they've developed, alternatives such as TCM, osteopathy, and naturopathy are often better options for achieving and preserving balanced health.

- This education must also include recognizing that the burden of reproductive health—which currently falls almost entirely on women, even when the issue is male factor infertility—should fall equally on men and women. This, too, requires broad public education to reduce stigma and allow men to talk about their fertility issues.
- Workplace policies should also address young couples who might be ready to start families earlier in their lives—but for the risk they will lose their place on the job track. That means building policies that support family-building at any stage of life by offering subsidized day care, flexible work hours, and telecommute options, as well as educational opportunities that allow employees with families and those experiencing fertility challenges to take advantage of career-building educational opportunities.

Maybe the rest of the world could follow the example of Norway,[4] where there is support in the workplace for family-building and where women and couples are provided with government support to continue their education while having infants. Maybe our culture should say, "Don't worry. You don't have to have a perfect life before having kids. There is no such thing as a perfect time and there certainly is no such thing as the 'perfect mate.'" More than anything, our culture should provide options that support women and men to have families while they're young and reproductively healthy but also support and monitor their reproductive health until they're older if that's what they prefer, and then support them to address any fertility challenges that arise, whether through Western or Eastern medicine, or preferably a balanced combination of the two.

We have a long way to go to get there, but as the Chinese philosopher Lao Tzu said in the Tao Te Ching,[5] the longest journey begins with a single step.

Final thoughts

Having surrendered to my pathway to pregnancy, I have been there, and I know how you feel first-hand. I walk beside you in your journey, not above you, and I hope that my company helps you feel a little less lonely.

My job is to make a meaningful impact in the lives of women and couples who come to me. I hope through this book, I have done that by showing you that there is no one-size-fits-all approach to fertility challenges, but there is one that's right for you.

Over two decades in practice, I've seen it all. Over and above the case studies in this book, I've seen physical anomalies like heart-shaped uterus, two uteruses, Asherman's syndrome, genetic factor infertility, and infertility related to diabetes and thyroid disorders. Telling every story is beyond the scope of this book, but I hope that somewhere in these pages you've found someone you can identify with or some advice that works for you.

Whether you are planning to have a family in the distant future, just starting out, or have been trying for years, remember that life's a journey and not a destination. Having a baby is not somewhere you get to. Instead of looking at your fertility journey as a treacherous mountain to be climbed, try seeing it as an opportunity to look within at the fertile valley you already are, a river bottom capable of receiving and nurturing life (to paraphrase one of my favourite mentors and my friend Dr. Randine Lewis, author of *The Infertility Cure*).[6]

I advise you to place less emphasis on:

- Trying to force a baby into your belly. You cannot control this. Instead, accept this as training for parenting, since it's an illusion to think you can have full control of your future children's actions.

- Your age, fertility statistics, or pathology, which focus your attention on the idea that there is something wrong with you.
- Your past disappointments and grief.

I suggest you focus more of your energy on:

- Embracing all of you, faults and all. Let go of your shame with a healthy dose of self-love.
- Nurturing healthy relationships around you, especially with your partner. The fertility journey can drive couples apart, so nourish your relationship with love, intimacy, respect, and open communication.
- Living in the present and staying true to yourself, recognizing your need for self-preservation rather than saying yes to everything and running yourself thin.
- Using the tips and advice throughout this book to decrease your stress levels, even if it's just by finding five minutes at a time when you can be in control, eat better, and live your life in a healthier way.
- Striving for balance rather than perfection, accepting that you are perfectly imperfect.

I am not suggesting you live in denial of a clear diagnosis. I am saying that your diagnosis can be a jumping-off point, an opportunity to become proactive on your fertility journey and with your overall health. You are a dynamically changing human being. You and your body can change with a renewed perspective. This is not about setting you up for false expectations. It's about giving you hope that when you combine the best of East and West, you can uncover possibilities you might never have expected.

With a little consistency and a lot of patience, perseverance, and persistence, you never know what miracles can come.

The child-free option

Before leaving you, I want to address one last point. This book is called *Pathways to Pregnancy*, and it focuses on supporting individuals and couples intent on building families through pregnancy to achieve their dream. Although I touched briefly on the option of adoption, and encourage my patients to consider it as a viable alternative, replete with its own particular joys and challenges, I have not touched on those individuals and couples who, after struggling with fertility challenges, choose to live child-free.

But I want to acknowledge them, because this too is a valid option. I don't believe in infertility, and I don't use the word. I believe there are many ways to live a fertile life. You can be an awesome aunt to your siblings' or friends' children. You can be a mother to your friends when that's what they need. You can be fertile and productive in the paid or unpaid work you do in the world, whether it is work with children or simply work that will leave the world a better place for children yet to come.

Procreation is a powerful drive, but if in the end you decide you do not want to continue that journey, whether because you're out of money, you can't stand the rollercoaster ride anymore, or you choose not to pursue the adoption option, it is still important to find balance in your own life and your own health. Just as TCM has helped many people find the inner balance to welcome a child, it can help you find the balance you need to continue living a productive and joyful life without a child.

Whatever pathway you choose, I believe TCM is there for you, and the most powerful way it can be there for you is when you take the best of both East and West and balance them. Whatever pathway you choose—to pregnancy, adoption, or child-free living—I wish you love and kindness on your journey. And I thank you for spending this portion of your journey with me.

Acknowledgements

Thank you to Maggie Langrick, my publisher at LifeTree Media; Paris Spence-Lang, her right-hand man; and my editors, Michelle MacAleese and Lynne Melcombe for their guidance, wisdom, and belief in this book, which is so close to my heart. Without a doubt, this book would not have come to life without their encouragement and expertise in the written word.

I am truly indebted to my patients, who are also my greatest teachers. They inspire me every day for the miracles they are and have become. A special thanks goes out to the women and couples who opened their hearts to share their fertility journeys through these pages. I am honoured to have been a part of their pathways to pregnancy.

Thanks to my village of friends, family, and practitioners, both Western and Eastern, who helped me to conceive Zoe and this book, who include:

Dr. Tom Hannam, Dr. Marjorie Dixon, Dr. Cliff Librach, Dr. Yaakov Bentov, Rosy Rosati, Jan Silverman, Rae Dolman, Fiona McCulloch (ND), David Bray, Emily Cheng Koh, Cary Rendek, Miriam Erlichman, Sue Malinowski, Andrea Thurton, Andrea Salmoran, Lauren Chau, and Bianca Estrela.

I want to especially thank my colleagues at ALIVE Holistic Health Clinic, David Liang, Tanya Smith, Aik Kim Heng, Shawn Gallagher, and Tina Torii, for contributing to this book and for their continued care for our patients (and me). Their commitment, empathy, and expertise kept my mind and heart at ease knowing that our patients had the best level of care, even when I was off having fertility treatments or writing this book.

I am indebted to Dr. Randine Lewis for being my mentor and inspiration. As a pioneer in the field of integrative medicine and fertility in North America and abroad, I am thankful to be a founding member of Clinical Excellence in Fertility Professionals. As such, my gratitude goes out to all of my colleagues, past and present, who played a role in my personal fertility journey and contributed to this book.

To my brothers, Casey and Robert; Robert's wife, Renee; and my nieces, Lucy and Stella: I am forever grateful to have your love and support every step of the way.

To my mother-in-law, Danielle, for teaching her son to be an equal partner in marriage, and in life, thank you.

To Etienne and Emilie, for being like Zoe's siblings, thank you.

I also wish to thank my dad for his creative spirit. He gave me strength to do and think outside the box. He taught me the three Ps of patience, perseverance, and persistence in life, as well as to "never pass" on life's opportunities.

Thanks to my mom for providing me the courage to share my story without shame in order to make a difference in the lives of others. I thank her also for loving Zoe as much as I do and being there to take care of me, Zoe, and our family since Zoe's birth.

My deepest gratitude goes to my husband, Jean-Louis, not only for walking beside me on our pathway to pregnancy but for tolerating my being an absentee wife as I spent countless nights pounding away at the computer. Thank you for being my rock and a loving dad, husband, and equal partner on our journey.

And last but not least, to my daughter, Zoe, who gave me the strength and drive to write this book even before she was born. Zoe, without you, this book would never have been conceived. I love you to the ends of this earth.

Abbreviations

AFC   Antral Follicle Count
AMH   Anti-Mullerian Hormone
ART   Assisted Reproductive Technology
CBT   Cognitive Behavioural Therapy
CCRM Colorado Clinic of Reproductive Medicine
CM   Cycle Monitoring
DE   Delayed Ejaculation
D&C   Dilation and Curettage
ED   Erectile Dysfunction
EFT   Emotional Freedom Technique
EMDR Eye Movement Desensitization and Reprocessing
FET   Frozen Embryo Transfer
FSH   Follicle Stimulating Hormone
GI   Glycemic Index
HSG   Hysterosalpingoram
ICSI   Intracytoplasmic Sperm Injection
IUI   Intrauterine Insemination
IVC   Intravaginal Culture Device
IVF   In Vitro Fertilization
LIT   Lymphocyte Immunization Therapy
LH   Luteinizing Hormone

MFI Male Factor Infertility
NK Natural Killer (cells)
OCP Oral Contraceptive Pills
OPK Ovulation Predictor Kit
OHSS Ovarian Hyperstimulation Syndrome
PESA Percutaneous Epididymal Sperm Aspiration
PGD Pre-Genetic Diagnosis
PGS Pre-Implantation Genetic Screening
POR Poor Ovarian Reserve
PCOS Polycystic Ovarian Syndrome
RE Reproductive Endrocrinologist
SCH Subchorionic Hemorrhage
STD Sexually Transmitted Diseases
STI Sexually Transmitted Infections
TCM Traditional Chinese Medicine
TESA Testicular Sperm Aspiration
TESE Testicular Sperm Extraction
TTC Trying To Conceive
TSH Thyroid Stimulating Hormone
TURP Transurethral Resection of the Prostate
UTI Urinary Tract Infection
5-HTP 5-Hydroxytryptophan

Glossary

Adhesions—a form of scar tissue, adhesions form as tissues and organs that should not be connected stick together.

Advanced maternal age—a medical reference to women over the age of thirty-five who want to give birth.

Androgens—male hormones.

Anejaculatory—a severe case of erectile dysfunction, where a man has never been able to ejaculate.

Anti-mullerian hormone (AMH)—a hormone secreted by the ova (immature eggs in a woman's ovaries), currently considered the best predictor of ovarian reserve (see poor ovarian reserve).

Antral follicles (AF)—eggs containing ovarian follicles.

Asherman's syndrome—A rare condition of uterine scarring primarily caused by surgery (D&C, see *dilation and curettage*), and to a lesser extent by severe pelvic infections.

Assisted reproductive technologies (ART)—technologies such as IUI and IVF that are used to assist any aspect of the reproductive process.

Autoimmune infertility—a condition in which a woman's immune system rejects an embryo or prevents implantation.

Azoospermia—an absence of sperm production.

Beta HCG—a pregnancy hormone produced by the cells of the implanted embryo.

Bisphenol-A (BPA)—an ingredient found in plastics and the linings of cans, which can exhibit hormonal properties not safe for pregnancy.

Blastocyst—a five-day-old multi-celled embryo.

Chemical pregnancy—a non-viable pregnancy that is detected only through a pregnancy test with no visible signs.

Cognitive behavioural therapy (CBT)—a type of therapy that teaches the patient how to control the way they interpret their environment.

Cortisol—a hormone associated with elevated stress levels, which may impede the body's ability to produce essential reproductive hormones.

Chromosomal translocation (AKA Robertsonian translocation)—a condition in which a piece of a chromosome breaks off and is moved onto another chromosome, resulting in structural chromosomal abnormalities.

Cycle monitoring—a procedure in which a fertility clinic uses blood work and ultrasound to track a woman's menstrual cycle to determine peak times for ovulation, intercourse, and conception.

Delayed ejaculation (DE)—a condition in which a man has a normal erection but is unable to ejaculate through sexual intercourse, or can only ejaculate with great difficulty.

Dilation and curettage (D&C)—a procedure to remove tissue from inside the uterus, such as after a fetus has died without miscarrying (called a *missed abortion*).

DNA fragmentation—a condition in which breaks exist in the sperm's genetic blueprint; while the sperm may be able to fertilize an egg, it may increase risk of miscarriage.

Down-regulation—a procedure during which doctors inhibit a woman's menstrual cycle to suppress the release of eggs. It is usually followed by stimulation of ovulation, with the goal of releasing more than one egg at a time and increasing chances of conception.

Ectopic pregnancy—a condition in which the fetus develops outside the uterus, typically in one of the fallopian tubes.

Emotional freedom technique (EFT)—a psychological therapy that might help a patient let go of negative subconscious beliefs to allow for physical and emotional healing.

Endometrium—the inner mucous lining of the uterus.

Erectile dysfunction (ED)—a condition in which a man is consistently unable to achieve or maintain an erection for sexual activity over a three-month period.

Epigenetic changes—genetic changes that occur due to environmental influences.

Eye movement desensitization and reprocessing (EMDR)—a psychological therapy that might help a patient let go of negative subconscious beliefs to allow for physical and emotional healing.

Follicle stimulating hormone (FSH)—a hormone released by the pituitary gland to stimulate the growth and maturation of follicles and the eggs within them.

Folliculogenesis—the development of an egg from a resting germ cell to an ovulating follicle.

Frozen embryo transfer (FET)—a procedure in which embryos harvested during a previous IVF cycle are frozen and then thawed before transfer to the uterus.

Glycemic index—a list that ranks foods according to their effect on blood glucose levels.

Hashimoto's disease—a condition in which the body attacks the thyroid gland, which is responsible for releasing many hormones into the body.

Hydrosalpinx—a condition in which the fallopian tubes are blocked by fluid; if both tubes are blocked by fluid, it's called *bilateral hydrosalpinx*.

Hypogonadism—a condition causing chronically low testosterone levels.

Hypothyroidism—a condition causing chronically low levels of thyroid hormones.

Hysterosalpingogram—a procedure in which a dye is shot through the vagina prior to an x-ray in order to see images in the uterus and fallopian tubes and check for abnormalities or pathologies.

Idiopathic—a pathology that appears to happen spontaneously, without an identifiable cause.

Incompetent cervix—a condition in which the cervix, which is normally closed during pregnancy, is open and thus may not retain a pregnancy.

Infertility—a condition in which a woman has been having unprotected intercourse for a year without conceiving.

Intracytoplasmic sperm injection (ICSI)—a test in which semen is studied under a microscope and healthy sperm are chosen for injection into mature eggs.

Intrauterine insemination (IUI)—a procedure in which a catheter is used to introduce washed sperm directly into the uterus.

Intrauterine ultrasound—see *transvaginal ultrasound*.

In vitro fertilization (IVF)—a procedure in which eggs that have been fertilized in a lab are introduced directly into the uterus.

Klinefelter syndrome—a genetic anomaly in which a man is born with an extra X chromosome (XXY instead of XY), causing sterility.

Low motility—a condition in which sperm has an impaired ability to swim.

Luteinizing hormone (LH)—a hormone that stimulates ripening of the egg and ovulation (release of the egg).

Lymphocyte immunization therapy (LIT)—a procedure in which a male's washed and extracted white blood cells are injected into the female's forearm, theoretically allowing the body's immune system to develop an antibody response so the female's immune system will recognize the embryo as "self" rather than an invader.

Myomectomy—a surgical procedure to remove uterine fibroids.

Nocebo effect—Latin for "I shall harm," referring to a situation in which a physician's words or actions have an unintentionally negative effect on a patient.

Orchitis—a condition in which swelling and inflammation of the testicles impedes sperm production.

Ova—immature egg.

Ovarian hyperstimulation syndrome (OHSS)—a condition in which the ovaries become swollen and painful from excessive hormone stimulation.

Ovarian reserve—the number and quality of eggs remaining in a woman's ovaries.

Ovulation predictor kit (OPK) —an over-the-counter kit available from any pharmacy that detects from a woman's urine when she is most fertile.

Oxidative stress—a condition in which toxins in the body (from smoking, pollution, and chemicals in food, for example) can damage cells (such as eggs and sperm) in much the same way metal can rust when exposed to air.

Pap smear—a procedure in which a speculum is inserted into the cervix, which is then swabbed and tested for cervical cancer and other diseases.

Parasympathetic nervous system—a system that controls the relaxation response in the body by slowing heart rate and relaxing blood vessels and muscles.

Percutaneous epididymal sperm aspiration (PESA)—a procedure in which a small needle is inserted into the vas deferens to grab healthy sperm from a man with poor sperm count, motility, or morphology.

Placebo effect—a condition in which a patient responds favourably to a benign medication or treatment, such as sugar pills, because they believe it will help.

Phthalates—a type of chemical that makes plastic soft and flexible but may be associated with toxicity affecting fertility.

Phytoestrogens—estrogens that occur naturally in certain plants, such as soy.

Polycystic ovarian syndrome (PCOS)—a condition of hormonal imbalance in which the ovaries develop cysts, and may make more androgens (male hormones) than normal, interfering with ovulation and menstruation.

Polyp—a benign growth that protrudes from a mucous membrane such as the uterus or a sinus.

Poor ovarian reserve (POR)—a condition in which the number and quality of eggs remaining in a woman's ovaries is considered to reflect poorly on her chances of conceiving with her own eggs.

Pre-implantation genetic screening (PGS)—a process of removing one cell from a day five or six embryo to be tested for genetic viability before it is transferred to the uterus.

Pre-washed sperm—a procedure in which normal, dense sperm are separated from semen and lighter, non-viable sperm using a centrifuge.

Retrograde ejaculation—a condition in which the semen goes backward into the bladder rather than out of the penis.

Robertsonian translocation—see *chromosomal translocation*.

Salpingectomy—a surgical procedure in which a fallopian tube is removed. If both tubes are removed, it's called a bilateral salpingectomy.

Secondary infertility—a condition in which a woman has difficulty conceiving a second child and carrying it to term, particularly after a first child has been conceived easily.

Septate uterus—a malformation in which the uterus is partially or fully divided by a wall (septum).

Sonohysterogram—a procedure in which a saltwater solution is injected into the uterus so it can be viewed through ultrasound to expose abnormalities that might contribute to miscarriage or difficulty conceiving.

Subchorionic hemorrhage—a condition in which blood pools between the embryo and the uterine wall in the womb.

Sub-fertile—a less than optimal state of fertility, but one in which there is still a chance of conceiving.

Superovulation—a procedure undertaken to stimulate the ovaries to create more than one egg, increasing the chance of conception.

T-Regulatory cells—cells that keep the immune system in check so it doesn't kill everything off.

Testicular Sperm Aspiration (TESA)—a procedure in which a small needle is inserted into the testicles to grab healthy sperm from a man with low sperm count, motility, or morphology.

Testicular Sperm Extraction (TESE)—a surgical procedure to isolate viable sperm by removing testicular tissue performed on men who have no sperm in their ejaculate.

Thrombophilia—a blood clotting issue that can impact fertility.

Transducer—a phallic-shaped probe inserted into the vagina during a trans-vaginal ultrasound.

Transurethral resection of the prostate (TURP)—prostate removal.

Trans-vaginal ultrasound—an ultrasound procedure in which a transducer is inserted into the vagina to create an image of the antral follicles and track follicular growth. Also called *intrauterine ultrasound*.

Trisomy 18—a chromosomal condition caused by an error in cell division that interferes with proper development, also known as Edwards syndrome.

Unexplained infertility—a term used when known causes for infertility have been explored and no medical explanation has been found.

Uterine fibroids—non-cancerous uterine tumours composed of dense, fibrous tissue.

Varicocele—a condition in which a varicose vein develops in the sperm cord, often visible on the scrotum.

White-coat hypertension (AKA white-coat syndrome)—a condition in which a patient who has normal blood pressure at home experiences an increase in blood pressure when tested in a clinical setting.

Xenoestrogens—environmental endocrine disruptors with estrogen-like effects.

Notes

1 YOU ARE NOT YOUR DIAGNOSIS

1   W.P. Kennedy, "The Nocebo Reaction," *Medical World,* 95 (1961): 203–205.

2   D. Johnston, Raising Expectations: Recommendations of the Expert Panel on Infertility and Adoption, Ontario Expert Panel on Infertility and Adoption; Ministry of Children and Youth Services, 2009.

3   R.W. Bretveld, C.M.G. Thomas, P.T.J. Scheepers, G.A. Zielhuis, and N. Roeleveld. "Pesticide Exposure: The Hormonal Function of the Female Reproductive System Disrupted?" Reprod Biol Endocrinol 4 (2006): 30.

4   T. Strünker, N. Goodwin, C. Brenker, et al., "The CatSper Channel Mediates Progesterone-Induced Ca2i Influx In Human Sperm. Nature 471 (2011): 382–386.

5   M.G. Enza, A. Cavallaro, T. Ainis,et al., "Anti-Inflammatory Effect of Lemon Mucilage: In Vivo and In Vitro Studies, Immunopharmacol Immunotoxicol 27 (2005): 661–70.

6   M.-A. Kim, J.-K. Sakong, E.-J. Kim, E.-H. Kim, and E.-H. Kim, "Effect of Aromatherapy Massage for the Relief of Constipation in the Elderly," Taehan Kanho Hakhoe Chi 35 (2005): 56–64.

7   K. Migiwa, T. Takeuchi, and E. Harada, "Lemon Oil Vapor Causes an Anti-Stress Effect via Modulating the 5-HT and DA Activities in Mice," Behav Brain Res 172 (2006): 240–9. Epub 15 Jun 2006.

8   Y. Fukuchi, M. Hiramitsu, M. Okada, et al., "Lemon Polyphenols Suppress Diet-Induced Obesity by Up-Regulation of mRNA Levels of the Enzymes Involved in Beta-Oxidation in Mouse White Adipose Tissue," *J Clin Biochem Nutr* 43 (2008): 201–209.

9   G.J. Song, E.P. Norkus, and V. Lewis. "Relationship between Seminal Ascorbic Acid and Sperm DNA Integrity in Infertile Men," International Journal of Andrology 29 (2006): 569–575.

10 S. Podzimek, "Sensitization to Inorganic Mercury Could Be a Risk Factor for Infertility," Neuroendocrinology Letters 26 (2005): 277–282.

11 K. Neeti and T. Prakash, "Effects of Heavy Metal Poisoning During Pregnancy," International Research Journal of Environment Sciences 2 (2013): 88–92.

12 C. Gundacker and M. Hengstschläger, "The Role of the Placenta in Fetal Exposure to Heavy Metals," Wiener Medizinische Wochenschrift Wien Med Wochenschr 162 (2012): 201–206.

13 P.M. Kidd, "Omega-3 DHA and EPA for Cognition, Behavior, and Mood: Clinical Findings and Structural-Functional Synergies with Cell Membrane Phospholipids," Altern Med Rev 12 (2007): 207–27.

14 M.R. Safarinejad, S.Y. Hosseini, F. Dadkhah, and M.A. Asgari, "Relationship of Omega-3 and Omega-6 Fatty Acids with Semen Characteristics, and Anti-Oxidant Status of Seminal Plasma: A Comparison between Fertile and Infertile Men," Clin Nutr 29 (2010): 100–105.

15 F. Hammiche, M. Vujkovic, W. Wijburg, et al., "Increased Preconception Omega-3 Polyunsaturated Fatty Acid Intake Improves Embryo Morphology," Fertil Steril 95 (2011): 1820–1823.

16 J.E. Chavarro, J.W. Rich-Edwards, B.A. Rosner, and W.C. Willett. "A Prospective Study of Dietary Carbohydrate Quantity and Quality in Relation to Risk of Ovulatory Infertility," Eur J Clin Nutr 63 (2011): 78–86.

17 S. Ahmed, K. Guillem, and Y. Valaele, "Sugar Addiction: Pushing the Drug-Sugar Analogy to the Limit," Curr Opin Clin Nutr Metab Care 16 (2013): 434–439.

18 J.E. Chavarro, W.C. Willett, and P.J. Skerrett, "The Fertility Diet: Groundbreaking Research Reveals Natural Ways to Boost Ovulation and Improve Your Chances of Getting Pregnant," J Clin Invest 118 (2008): 1210.

19 A. Odegaard and M.A. Pereira, "Trans Fatty Acids, Insulin Resistance, and Type 2 Diabetes," Nutr Rev, 64 (2006): 364–72.

20 F.L.P. Soares, R. de Oliveira Matoso, L.G. Teixeira, et al., "Gluten-Free Diet Reduces Adiposity, Inflammation and Insulin Resistance Associated with the Induction of PPAR-Alpha and PPAR-Gamma Expression," J Nutr Biochem 24 (2013): 1105–1111.

21 U. Volta and V. Villanacci. "Celiac Disease: Diagnostic Criteria in Progress," Cell Molecular Immunol 8 (2011): 96–102; Epub 31 January 2011.

22 EWG, Shopper's Guide to Pesticides in Produce (2016), http://www.ewg.org/foodnews/list.php.

23 J.S. Tolstrup, S.K. Kjær, C. Holst, et al., "Alcohol Use as Predictor for Infertility in a Representative Population of Danish Women," Acta Obstetricia et Gynecologica Scandinavica 82 (2003): 744–749.

24 X. Weng , R. Odouli, and D.K. Li, "Maternal Caffeine Consumption during Pregnancy and the Risk of Miscarriage: A Prospective Cohort Study," Am J Obstet Gynecol 198 (2008);198: 279.e1–8.

25 T. Crozier, A. Stalmach, M. Lean, and A. Crozier. "Espresso Coffees, Caffeine and Chlorogenic Acid Intake: Potential Health Implications," Food and Function 3 (2012): 30–33.

26 M. Szewczuk, "Polymorphism of the Insulin-Like Growth Factor 1 Receptor Gene (IGF1R/e10/MspI and IGF1R/e16/RsaI) in Four Dairy Breeds and its Association with Milk Traits," Livestock Science 181 (2015): 43–50.

27 R. Mora-Ripoll, "The Therapeutic Value of Laughter in Medicine," Altern Ther Health Med 16 (2010): 56–64.

28 T. Crozier, A. Stalmach, M. Lean, and A. Crozier. "Espresso Coffees, Caffeine and Chlorogenic Acid Intake: Potential Health Implications," Food and Function 3 (2012): 30–33.

29 Bureau of Labor Statistics, United States Department of Labor, "1901," http://www.bls.gov/opub/uscs/1901.pdf.

2 THE EVERYWOMAN OF FERTILITY CHALLENGES

1   B.H. Lipton, The Biology of Belief: Unleashing the Power of Consciousness, Matter, and Miracles (Santa Rosa, CA: Hay House, 2005), p. 15.

2   A. Shrim, S.E. Elizur, D.S. Seidman, J. Rabinovici, A. Wiser, and J. Dor, "Elevated Day 3 FSH/ LH Ratio Due to Low LH Concentration Predicts Reduced Ovarian Response," Reprod Bio Medicine 12 (2006): 418–422.

3   J. Johnson, J. Canning, T. Kaneko, J. Pru, and J.L. Tilly, "Germline Stem Cells and Follicular Renewal in the Postnatal Mammalian Ovary," Nat Med Nature Medicine 428 (2004):145–150.

4   Y. White, D.C. Woods, Y. Takai, O. Ishihara, H. Seki, and J.L. Tilly, "Oocyte Formation by Mitotically Active Germ Cells Purified from Ovaries of Reproductive-Age Women," Nat Med Nature Medicine 18 (2012): 413–421.

5   A. Iwase, T. Nakamura, S. Osuka, S. Takikawa, M. Goto, and F. Kikkawa. "Anti-Müllerian Hormone as a Marker of Ovarian Reserve: What Have We Learned, and What Should We Know?" Repro Med Biol (2015): 1–10.

6   C. Goldin and L.F. Katz, "The Power of the Pill: Oral Contraceptives and Women's Career and Marriage Decisions," Journal of Political Economy 110 (2002):730–770.

7   A. Sonfield, K. Hasstedt, M.L. Kavanaugh, and R. Anderson, The Social and Economic Benefits of Women's Ability to Determine Whether and When to Have Children (Guttmacher Institute, USA: 2013), pp. 11–16. http://www.demonish.com/cracker/1431519197_7cf1db0374/social-economic-benefits.pdf.

8   Bureau of Labor Statistics, United States Department of Labor, Current Population Survey, 2013 (from Table 2, "Employment Status of the Civilian Noninstitutional Population 16 Years and Over by Sex, 1972 to Date").

9   United States Census Bureau, "DataFerrett," *Current Population Survey*,
    Monthly Microdata, December 2014.
10 Statistics Canada, "Labour Force Characteristics by Sex and Age Group," 2012.
11 United States Census Bureau, "DataFerrett," *Current Population Survey*,
    Monthly Microdata, December 2014.

3   MORE THAN SURVIVING

1   K. Wisner, D. Sit, B. Hanusa, et al., "Major Depression and Antidepressant
    Treatment: Impact on Pregnancy and Neonatal Outcomes," Am J Psychiatry
    7 (2009), 557–566.
2   A. Domar, P.C. Zuttermeister, and R. Friedman, "The Psychological Impact
    of Infertility: A Comparison with Patients with Other Medical Conditions,"
    J Psychosom Obstet Gynaecol 14 (1993): 45–52.
3   L. Eshkevari, R. Egan, D. Phillips, et al., "Acupuncture at St36 Prevents
    Chronic Stress-Induced increases in neuropeptide Y in rat," Exp Biol
    Medicine 237 (2012): 18–23.
4   American Society for Reproductive Medicine, "PCOS: Is the Pill the Only
    Answer?" (from Question 2, "How Do I Know if I Could Benefit from
    Psychological Counseling?" http://www.asrm.org/search/detail.aspx?id=-
    2356&q=depression%20and%20infertility.
5   Public Health Agency of Canada, "What are the Symptoms of Depression?"
    http://www.phac-aspc.gc.ca/cd-mc/mi-mm/depression-eng.php.
6   R. Jerath, J.W. Edry, V.A. Barnes, and V. Jerath, "Physiology of Long
    Pranayamic Breathing: Neural Respiratory Elements May Provide a
    Mechanism that Explains How Slow Deep Breathing Shifts the Autonomic
    Nervous System," Medical Hypotheses 67 (2006): 566–571.
7   R.E. Anglin, Z. Samaan, S.D. Walter, and S.D. McDonald, "Vitamin D
    Deficiency and Depression in Adults: Systematic Review and Meta-Analysis,"
    Br J Psychiatry 202 (2013):100–107.
8   G. Resler, R. Lavie, J. Campos, et al., "Effect of Folic Acid Combined with
    Fluoxetine in Patients with Major Depression on Plasma Homocysteine and
    Vitamin B12, and Serotonin Levels in Lymphocytes,"
    Neuroimmunomodulation 15 (2008): 145–152.
9   S. Hanna, L. Lachover, and R. P. Rajarethinam, "Vitamin B12 Deficiency and
    Depression in the Elderly: Review and Case Report," Prim Care Companion
    J Clin Psychiatry 11 (2009): 269–270.
10 M. Morgese, P. Tucci, E. Mhillaj, et al., "Lifelong Nutritional Omega-3
    Deficiency Evokes Depressive-Like State through Soluble Beta Amyloid,"
    Mol Neurobiol (2016 Feb 29, Epub ahead of print).

11 K.A. Shaw, J. Turner, and C. Del Mar, "Tryptophan and 5-Hydroxytryptophan for Depression," Cochrane Database Syst Rev (2002), http://dx.doi.org/10.1002/14651858.CD003198.

12 H. MacPherson, S. Richmond, M. Bland, et al., "Acupuncture and Counselling for Depression in Primary Care: A Randomised Controlled Trial," PLOS Medicine 10.1371/journal.pmed.1001518, (Sep 2013).

13 Y. Zhang, M. Han, Z. Liu, J. Wang, Q He, and J. Liu, "Chinese Herbal Formula Xiao Yao San for Treatment of Depression: A Systematic Review of Randomized Controlled Trials," Evid Based Complement Alternat Med (2012) 2012:931636, doi: 10.1155/2012/931636, Epub 22 Aug 2011.

14 A.D.A.C. Smith, K. Tilling, S.M. Nelson, D.A. Lawlor. "Live-Birth Rate associated with Repeat In Vitro Fertilization Treatment Cycles," JAMA 314 (December 22/29, 2015).

15 Ibid.

16 T. Lee, Z. Zheng, "Acupuncture Pain Research: Quantitative and Qualitative," Acupuncture for Pain Management, (Springer: 11 September 2013): 117–137.

17 A.J. Vickers, D. Phil, and K. Linde, "Acupuncture for Chronic Pain," JAMA 311 (2014): 955–956, doi:10.1001/jama.2013.285478.

18 L. Eshkevari, R. Egan, D. Phillips, et al., "Acupuncture at St36 Prevents Chronic Stress-Induced increases in neuropeptide Y in rat," Exp Biol Medicine 237 (2012): 18–23.

19 L.H. Rubin, M. Opsahl, K. Wiemer, S. Mist, and A. Caughey, "Impact of Whole Systems Traditional Chinese Medicine on In-Vitro Fertilization Outcomes," Reprod BioMed Online 30 (2015): 602–612.

20 S. Jackson and K.W. Singletary, "Sulforaphane Inhibits Human MCF-7 Mammary Cancer Cell Mitotic Progression and Tubulin Polymerization," J Nutrition 134 (2004): 2229–2236.

21 A. Ackerson, "Milk Thistle," Better Nutrition 68 (2006): 8–9.

22 K. Wisner, D. Sit, B. Hanusa, E. Moses-Kolko, D. Bogen, D. Hunker, and L. Singer, "Major Depression and Antidepressant Treatment: Impact on Pregnancy and Neonatal Outcomes," Am J Psychiatry 7 (2009), 557–566.

4   DOING MORE IS NOT ALWAYS DOING BETTER

1 Centre for Disease Control and Prevention, Assisted Reproductive Technology National Summary Report 2012, (2014): 20–21.

2 Practice Committee of the American Society for Reproductive Medicine, "Evaluation and treatment of Recurrent Pregnancy Loss: A Committee Opinion," Fertil Steril 98 (2012):1103–1111, doi: 10.1016.

3 K. Hurt, M. Guile, J. Beinstock, H. Fox, and E. Wallach, "Miscarriage and Recurrent Pregnancy Loss," Johns Hopkins Manual of Gynecology and Obstetrics, 4th ed. (Wolters Kluwer, USA: 2011), p. 438.

4 C. Garrido-Gimenez and J. Alijotas-Reig, "Recurrent Miscarriage: Causes, Evaluation and Management," Postgrad Med J 91 (2015):151–162, doi:10.1136/postgradmedj-2014–132672.

5 A. Stagnaro-Green, "Thyroid Antibodies and Miscarriage: Where Are We at a Generation Later?" J Thyroid Res (2011), Article ID 841949, doi:10.4061/2011/841949.

6 D.K. Tobias, S.A. Missmer, F.B. Hu, et al., "History of Infertility and Risk of Type 2 Diabetes Mellitus: A Prospective Cohort Study," Diabetologia 58 (2015): 707–15. Epub 18 Jan 2015.

7 G. Toft, Bo A.G Jönsson, C.H. Lindh, et al. "Association between Pregnancy Loss and Urinary Phthalate Levels around the Time of Conception," Environ Health Perspect 120 (2012): 458–463.

8 R.B. Lathi, K.F. Brookfield, V.L. Baker, et al., "Conjugated Bisphenol A in Maternal Serum in Relation to Miscarriage Risk," Fertil Steril 102 (2014):123–128.

9 K. Neeti and T. Prakash, "Effects of Heavy Metal Poisoning during Pregnancy," Int Res J Environ Sci 2 (2013): 88–92.

10 S. Friedler, S. Glasser, L. Azani, et al., "The Effect of Medical Clowning on Pregnancy Rates after In Vitro Fertilization and Embryo Transfer," Fertil Steril 95 (2011): 2127–30.

11 K. Wisner, D. Sit, B. Hanusa, et al., "Major Depression and Antidepressant Treatment: Impact on Pregnancy and Neonatal Outcomes," Am J Psychiatry 7 (2009), 557–566.

12 B. Grajewski, "Miscarriages Amongst Flight Attendants Background: Cosmic Radiation and Circadian Disruption are Potential Reproductive Hazards for Flight Attendants," Epidemiology 26 (2015):192–203.

5 THE MALE FACTOR

1 Resolve: The National Infertility Association (USA), "Male Workup: The Semen Analysis," http://www.resolve.org/about-infertility/male-workup/the-semen-analysis.html?referrer=https://www.google.ca/.

2 American Society for Reproductive Medicine, Report on Varicocele and Infertility, Fertil Steril 90 (Suppl 3), (2008): S247–S249.

3 B.K. Canales, D.M. Zapzalka, C.J. Ercole, et al., "Prevalence and Effect of Varicoceles in an Elderly Population," Urology 66 (2005): 627–631.

4 P. Kanagarajah, R. Ayyathurai, and C.M. Lynne, "Male Infertility and Adult Polycystic Kidney Disease—Revisited: Case Report and Current Literature Review," Andrologia 44 (2012): 838–841.

5 G. Anifandis, T. Bounartzi, C.I. Messini, K. Dafopoulos, S. Sotiriou, and I.E. Messini, "The Impact of Cigarette Smoking and Alcohol Consumption on Sperm Parameters and Sperm DNA Fragmentation (SDF) Measured by Halosperm," Arch Gynecol Obstet 290 (2014): 777–82.

6 L. Whan, N. Mcclure, and S. Lewis, "Effects of Delta-9-Tetrahydrocannabinol, the Primary Psychoactive Cannabinoid In Marijuana, on Human Sperm Function In Vitro," Fertil Steril 85 (2005), 653–660, doi:10.1016/j.fertnstert.2005.08.027.

7 M.F. Elshal, I.H. El-Sayed, M.A. Elsaied, S.A. El-Masry, and T.A. Kumosani, "Sperm Head Defects and Disturbances in Spermatozoal Chromatin and DNA Integrities in Idiopathic Infertile Subjects: Association with Cigarette Smoking," Clin Biochem 42 (2009): 589–594.

8 S. Belloc, M. Cohen-Bacrie, E. Amar, et al., "High Body Mass Index Has a Deleterious Effect on Semen Parameters Except Morphology: Results from a Large Cohort Study," Fertil Steril 102 (2014):1268–73, doi: 10.1016/j.fertnstert.2014.07.1212, Epub 12 Sep 2014.

9 S. La Vignera, R. Condorelli, E. Vicari, R. D'Agata, and A.E. Calogero, "Diabetes Mellitus and Sperm Parameters," J of Andrology 3 (2013).

10 Y. Shynkin, M. Jung, P. Yoo, D. Schulsinger, and E. Komaroff, "Laptop Computers (LC) & Cell Phones. Increase in Scrotal Temperature in Laptop Computer Users," Hum Reprod 20 (2005): 452–455.

11 A. Garolla, M. Torino, B. Sartini, et al., "Seminal and Molecular Evidence that Sauna Exposure affects Human Spermatogenesis," Hum Reprod 28 (2013): 877–885.

12 J. Jurewicz, M. Radwan, W. Sobala, et al., "Lifestyle Factors and Sperm Aneuploidy," Reprod Biol 14 (2014):190–9, doi: 10.1016/j.repbio.2014.02.002, Epub 4 Mar 2014.

13 L. De-Kun, Z. ZhiJun, M. Maohua, et al., "Urine Bisphenol-A (BPA) Level in Relation to Semen Quality," Fertil Steril 95 (2011): 625–630.

14 The Doctors Laboratory, "Information about Sperm DNA Fragmentation," http://www.tdlpathology.com/services-divisions/tdl-andrology/sperm-dna-fragmentation.

15 The Turek Clinic, "It Takes Two to Tango," http://theturekclinic.com/two-to-tango-sperm-egg-miscarriages-male-infertility/.

16 D. Johnston, Raising Expectations: Recommendations of the Expert Panel on Infertility and Adoption, Ontario Expert Panel on Infertility and Adoption; Ministry of Children and Youth Services, 2009, p. 89.

17 A.J. Gaskins, D.S. Colaci, J. Mendiola, S.H. Swan, and J.E. Chavarro, "Dietary Patterns and Semen Quality in Young Men," Hum Reprod 27 (2012):2899–907, doi: 10.1093/humrep/des298. Epub 12 Aug 2012.

18 A. Cutillas-Tolin, L. Minguez-Alarcon, J. Mendiola, et al., "Mediterranean and Western Dietary Patterns are Related to Markers of Testicular Function among Healthy Men," Hum Reprod 25 (2015), pii: dev236.

19 M. Afeiche, P.L. Williams, J. Mendiola, et al., "Dairy Food Intake in Relation to Semen Quality and Reproductive Hormone Levels among Physically Active Young Men," Hum Reprod 28 (2013):2265–75, doi: 10.1093/humrep/det133, Epub 12 May 2013.

20 L.I. Kolesnikova, S.I., Kolesnikov, N.A. Kurashova, and T.A. Bairova, "Causes and Factors of Male Infertility," Vestnik Rossiiskoi Akademii Meditsinskikh Nauk 70 (2015): 579–584.

21 K. Muthusami and P. Chinnaswamy, "Effect of Chronic Alcoholism on Male Fertility Hormones and Semen Quality," Fertil Steril 84 (2005): 919–924, doi:10.1016/j.fertnstert.2005.04.025.

22 J. Jurewicz, M. Radwan, S. Wojciech, et al., "Lifestyle and Semen Quality: Role Of Modifiable Risk Factors," Syst Biol Reprod Med 60 (2014): 43–51.

23 T. Janevic, L.G. Kahn, P. Landsbergis, et al., "Effects of Work and Life Stress on Semen Quality," Fertil Steril 102 (2014) :530–538, doi: 10.1016/j.fertnstert.2014.04.021, Epub 23 May 2014.

24 Ibid.

25 C. Wright, S. Milne, and H. Leeson, "Sperm DNA Damage Caused by Oxidative Stress: Modifiable Clinical, Lifestyle and Nutritional Factors in Male Infertility," Reprod BioMed Online 28 (2014): 684–703.

26 S.O. Hamouda, J. Perrin, V. Achard, et al., "Association between Sperm Abnormalities and Occupational Environment Among Male Consulting for Couple Infertility," J Gynecol Obstet Biol Reprod 45 (2016):1–10, doi: 10.1016/j.jgyn.2015.08.011, Epub 19 Sep 2015.

27 A. Garolla, M. Torino, B. Sartini, et al., "Seminal and Molecular Evidence that Sauna Exposure Affects Human Spermatogenesis," Hum Reprod 28 (2013): 877–885.

28 Y. Shynkin, M. Jung, P. Yoo, D. Schulsinger, and E . Komaroff, "Laptop Computers (LC) & Cell Phones. Increase in Scrotal Temperature in Laptop Computer Users," Hum Reprod 20 (2005): 452–455.

29 R. Rago, P. Salacone, L. Caponecchia, et al., "The Semen Quality of the Mobile Phone Users," J Endocrinol Invest 36 (2013): 970–974; A. Agarwal, F. Deepinder, R.K. Sharma, G. Ranga, and J. Li , "Effect of Cell Phone Usage on Semen Analysis in Men Attending Infertility Clinic: An Observational Study," Fertil Steril 89 (2008): 124–128); T. Gutschi, B. Mohamad, R. Shamloul, K. Pummer, and H. Trummer, "Impact of Cell Phone Use on Men's Semen Parameters," Andrologia 43 (2011): 312–316.

30 J. Jurewicz, M. Radwan, W. Sobala, et al., "Lifestyle Factors and Sperm Aneuploidy," Reprod Biol 14 (2014):190–9, doi: 10.1016/j.repbio.2014.02.002, Epub 4 Mar 2014.

31 N. Whator, K. Umeizudike, P. Avanbadejo, et al., Another Reason for Impeccable Oral Hygiene: Oral Hygiene-Sperm Count Link," *J Contemp Dent Pract* 15 (20143): 352–358.

32 P. Turek, "Male Fertility and Infertility: Medications and Toxins," http://theturekclinic.com/services/male-fertility-infertility-doctor-treatments-issues-zero-sperm-count-male-doctors/non-surgical-male-fertility-infertility-causes-treatment/.

33 R. Sharma, A. Agarwal, V.K. Rohra, M. Assidi, M. Abu-Elmagd, and R.F. Turki, "Effects of Increased Paternal Age on Sperm Quality, Reproductive Outcome and Associated Epigenetic Risks to Offspring," Reprod Biol Endocrinol 13 (2015):35, doi: 10.1186/s12958-015-0028-x.

34 R.P. Smith and P.J. Turek, "Sperm and Ejaculation. Netter Collection of Medical Illustrations: Reproductive System," Section 5: 99–108.

35 J.P. Curley, R. Mashoodh, and F.A. Champagne, "Epigenetics and the Origins of Paternal Effects," Horm Behav 59 (2011): 306–314.

36 B.F. Hales and B. Robaire, "Paternal Exposure to Drugs and Environmental Chemicals: Effects on Progeny Outcome," J Androl 22 (2001): 927–936.

37 L.M. Anderson, L. Riffle, R. Wilson, G.S. Travlos, M.S. Lubomirski, and W.G. Alvord, "Preconceptional Fasting of Fathers Alters Serum Glucose in Offspring of Mice," Nutrition 22 (2006): 327–331.

38 Weill Cornell Medical College, James Buchanan Brady Foundation, Department of Urology, https://www.cornellurology.com/clinical-conditions/male-infertility/general-information/lifestyle/

39 E. Greco, M. Iacobelli, L. Rienzi, F. Ubaldi, S. Ferrero, and J Tesarik, "Reduction of the Incidence of Sperm DNA Fragmentation by Oral Antioxidant Treatment," J Andrology 26 (2005).

40 X. Zhou, F. Liù, and S. Zhai. "Effect of L-carnitine and/or L-acetyl-carnitine in Nutrition Treatment for Male Infertility: A Systematic Review," Asia Pacific J Clin Nutr 16 Suppl 1 (2007): 383–390.

41 Y.J. Menezo, A. Hazout, G. Panteix,et al., "Antioxidants to Reduce Sperm DNA Fragmentation: An Unexpected Adverse Effect," Reprod Biomed Online 14 (2007): 418–421.

42 C. Abad, M.J. Amengual, J. Gosalvez, et al., "Effects of Oral Antioxidant Treatment upon the Dynamics of Human Sperm DNA Fragmentation and Subpopulations of Sperm with Highly Degraded DNA," Andrologia 45 (2013): 211–216.

43 Weill Cornell Medical College, James Buchanan Brady Foundation, Department of Urology, https://www.cornellurology.com/clinical-conditions/ male-infertility/general-information/lifestyle/

44 G. Azizollahi, S. Azizollahi, H. Babaei, et al., "Effects of Supplement Therapy on Sperm Parameters, Protamine Content and Acrosomal Integrity of Varicocelectomized Subjects," *J Assist Reprod Genet* 30 (2013): 593–599.

45 C. Abad, M.J. Amengual, J. Gosalvez, et al., "Effects of Oral Antioxidant Treatment upon the Dynamics of Human Sperm DNA Fragmentation and Subpopulations of Sperm with Highly Degraded DNA," Andrologia 45 (2013): 211–216.

46 K. Tremellen, G. Miari, D. Froiland, and J. Thompson, "A Randomised Control Trial Examining the Effect of an Antioxidant (Menevit) on Pregnancy Outcome During IVF-ICSI Treatment," Aust. N. Z. J. Obstet. Gynaecol 47 (2007): 216–221.

47 G. Corona, E. Mannucci, L. Petrone, et al., "Psychobiological Correlates of Delayed Ejaculation in Male Patients With Sexual Dysfunctions," J Androl 27 (2006): 453–458.

48 Mayo Clinic, http://www.mayoclinic.org/diseases-conditions/delayed-ejaculation/ basics/causes/con-20034981

49 Medline Plus, "Delayed Ejaculation: Causes,"https://www.nlm.nih.gov/ medlineplus/ency/article/001954.htm

50 J. Morton, "Hug Me," The Sydney Sun-Herald, Feb 14, 2016.

51 I. A. Aytac,, J. B. McKinlay, and R. J. Krane, "The Likely Worldwide Increase in Erectile Dysfunction between 1995 and 2025 and Some Possible Policy Consequences," BJU International 84 (1999): 50–56.

52 E. Selvin, A.L. Burnett, and E. Platz, "Prevalence and Risk Factors for Erectile Dysfunction in the US," Am J Med 120 (2007):151–157.

53 Ibid.

54 V. Soni, A.W. Pastuszak, M. Khera, "Erectile Dysfunction and Infertility," Men's Sexual Health and Fertility: A Clinician's Guide, 89–90.

55 A.M. Landtblom, "Treatment of Erectile Dysfunction in Multiple Sclerosis," Expert Rev Neurother 6 (2006):931–935.

6 MAKING THE WORKPLACE WORK FOR FERTILITY

1 R.S. Legro, S.A. Arslanian, D.A. Ehrmann, et al., "Diagnosis and Treatment of Polycystic OvarySyndrome: An Endocrine Society Clinical Practice Guideline," J Clin Endocrinol Metab 98 (2013):4565–92, doi: 10.1210/jc.2013-2350.

2 S. Franks, Polycystic Ovary Syndrome, N Engl J Med 333 (1995): 853–861.

3 J. Mehta, V. Kamdar, and D. Dumesic, "Phenotypic Expression of Polycystic Ovary Syndrome in South Asian Women," Obstet Gynecol Surv 68 (2013): 228–234, doi: 10.1097/OGX.0b013e318280a30f.

4   F. McCulloch. *8 Steps to Reverse Your PCOS: A Proven Program to Reset Your Hormones, Repair Your Metabolism, and Restore Your Fertility.* Austin, TX: Greenleaf Book Group Press; 2016.

5   J. Cedernaes, H.B. Schiöth, and C. Benedict, "Determinants of Shortened, Disrupted, and Mistimed Sleep and Associated Metabolic Health Consequences in Healthy Humans," Diabetes 64 (2015): 1073–1080.

6   E.S. Ford, C. Li, A.G. Wheaton, D.P. Chapman, G.S. Perry, and J.B. Croft, "Sleep Duration and Body Mass Index and Waist Circumference among U.S. Adults," *Obesity* 22 (2014):598–607.

7   X. Kang, L. Jia, and X. Shen, "Manifestation of Hyperandrogenism in the Continuous Light Exposure-Induced PCOS Rat Model," BioMed Res Int (2015), doi: 10.1155/2015/943694, Epub 3 May 2015.

8   A. Swanton, L. Storey, E. McVeigh, and T. Child, "IVF Outcome in Women with PCOS, PCO and Normal Ovarian Morphology," Eur J Obstet Gynecol Reprod Biol 149 (2010): 68–71, doi: 10.1016/j.ejogrb.2009.11.017, Epub 22 Dec 2009.

9   J. Johansson, L. Redman, P.P. Veldhuis, et al., "Acupuncture for Ovulation Induction in Polycystic Ovary Syndrome: A Randomized Controlled Trial," Am J Physiol Endocrinol Metab 304 (2013), doi: 10.1152/ajpendo.00039.2013.

10 R. Lewis, The Infertility Cure (New York: Little, Brown and Company, 2004) pp. 88–89.

11 D. Johnston, Raising Expectations: Recommendations of the Expert Panel on Infertility and Adoption, Ontario Expert Panel on Infertility and Adoption; Ministry of Children and Youth Services, 2009.

12 D.F. Halpern, "How Time-Flexible Work Policies Can Reduce Stress, Improve Health, and Save Money," Stress and Health 21 (2005):157–168.

13 K. Matos and E. Galinsky, "When Work Works. Workplace Flexibility in the United States: A Status Report," (USA: Families and Work Institute, 2011) pp. 22–23.

7   MAKING THE IMPOSSIBLE POSSIBLE

1   M.T.M. Franssen, J.C. Korevaar, F. van der Veen, N.J. Leschot, P.M. M. Bossuyt, M. Goddijn, "Reproductive Outcome After Chromosome Analysis in Couples with Two or More Miscarriages: Case-Control Study," BMJ 332 (2006): 759.

2   R.L. Bick, J. Madden, K.B. Heller, A. Toofanian. "Recurrent Miscarriage: Causes, Evaluation, and Treatment," Medscape General Medicine 1 (1998).

3   T. Nonaka, I. Ooki, T. Enomoto, and K. Takakuwa, "Complex Chromosomal Rearrangements in Couples Affected by Recurrent Spontaneous Abortion," Int J Gynaecol Obstet 128 (2015):36–39, doi: http://dx.doi.org/10.1016/j.ijgo.2014.07.018.

4   Ibid.

5   A.E. Beer and J. Kantecki, Is Your Body Baby Friendly?: Unexplained Infertility, Miscarriage, and IVF Failure Explained, (AJR Publishing: 2006) pp.141–155.

6   Ibid.

7   Ibid.

8   Ibid., p.4.

9   B.H. Lipton, The Biology of Belief: Unleashing the Power of Consciousness, Matter, and Miracles (Santa Rosa, CA: Hay House, 2005), p. 15.

10 Ibid. p. 135.

11 E. Stener-Victorin and X. Wu, "Effects and Mechanisms of Acupuncture in the Reproductive System," Autonomic Neuroscience 157 (2010): 46–51.

12 M. Cabyoglu, N. Ergene, and U. Tan, "The Mechanism of Acupuncture and Clinical Applications," Int J Neuroscience 116 (2006): 115–125.

13 Succeed Magazine, "Mind, Growth, and Matter," (interview with Bruce Lipton), June 7, 2012, https://www.brucelipton.com/resource/interview/mind-growth-and-matter.

14 E. Levitas, A. Parmet, E. Lunenfeld, Y. Bentov, E. Burstein, M. Friger, and G. Potashnik, "Impact of Hypnosis during Embryo Transfer on the Outcome of In Vitro Fertilization–Embryo Transfer: A Case-Control Study," Fertil Steril 85 (2006): 1404–1408.

15 A. Mendelsohn, Y. Chalamish, A. Solomonovich, and Y. Dudai, "Mesmerizing Memories: Brain Substrates of Episodic Memory Suppression in Posthypnotic Amnesia," Neuron 57 (2008): 159–170.

16 D. Chopra, Unconditional Life: Discovering the Power to Fulfill Your Dreams, (New York: Bantam Books, 1992) p. 245.

8   "THIS CAN'T BE HAPPENING TO ME"

1   A. Domar, P.C. Zuttermeister, and R. Friedman, "The Psychological Impact of Infertility: A Comparison with Patients with Other Medical Conditions," J Psychosom Obstet Gynaecol 14 (1993): 45–52.

2   S. Gaikwad, N. Garrido, A. Cobo, A. Pellicer, and J. Remohi, "Bed Rest after Embryo Transfer Negatively Affects In Vitro Fertilization: A Randomized Controlled Clinical Trial," Fertil Steril 100 (2013): 729–735.

3   K.P. Tremellen, D. Valbuena, J. Landeras, et al., "The Effect of Intercourse on Pregnancy Rates During Assisted Human Reproduction," Hum Reprod 15 (2000): 2653–2658.

4   G. Crawford, A. Ray, A. Gudi, A. Shah, and R. Homburg, "The Role of Seminal Plasma for Improved Outcomes during In Vitro Fertilization Treatment: Review Of The Literature And Meta-Analysis," Hum Reprod 21 (2015): 275–284.

5   S. Friedler, S. Glasser, L. Azani, et al., "The Effect of Medical Clowning on Pregnancy Rates after In Vitro and Embryo Transfer," Fertil Steril 95 (2011): 2127–2130.

6   W.E. Paulus, M. Zhang, E. Strehler, I. El-Danasouri, and K. Sterzik, "Influence of Acupuncture on the Pregnancy Rate in Patients Who Undergo Assisted Reproduction Therapy," Fertil Steril 77 (2002): 721–724.

9   MILLION-DOLLAR BABIES

1   W.E. Paulus, M. Zhang, E. Strehler, I. El-Danasouri, and K. Sterzik, "Influence of Acupuncture on the Pregnancy Rate in Patients Who Undergo Assisted Reproduction Therapy," Fertil Steril 77 (2002): 721–724.

2   B. Kok, K. Coffey, M. Cohn, et al., "How Positive Emotions Build Physical Health: Perceived Positive Social Connections Account for the Upward Spiral Between Positive Emotions and Vagal Tone," Psychol Sci 24 (2013): 1123–1132.

3   I. Gordona, O. Zagoory-Sharona, J.F. Leckmanc, and R. Feldman, "Oxytocin and the Development of Parenting in Humans," Biol Psychiatry 68 (2010): 377–382.

4   B. Ditzen, M. Schaer, B. Gabriel, G. Bodenmann, U. Ehlert, and M. Heinrichs, "Intranasal Oxytocin Increases Positive Communication and Reduces Cortisol Levels During Couple Conflict," Biol Psychiatry 65 (2009): 728–731.

5   M. Roque, M. Valle, F. Guimarães, M. Sampaio, and S. Geber, "Freeze-All Policy: Fresh Vs. Frozen-Thawed Embryo Transfer," Fertil Steril 103 (2015): 1190–1193.

6   A.D.A.C. Smith, K. Tilling, S.M. Nelson, and D.A. Lawlor, "Live-Birth Rate Associated with Repeat In Vitro Fertilization Treatment Cycles," JAMA 314 (2015), jama.jamanetwork.com.

7   D. Johnston, Raising Expectations: Recommendations of the Expert Panel on Infertility and Adoption, Ontario Expert Panel on Infertility and Adoption; Ministry of Children and Youth Services, 2009.

10   FEMALE-ONLY PREGNANCY

1   A. Rotkirch, "All That She Wants Is A(nother) Baby'? Longing for Children as a Fertility Incentive of Growing Importance," Journal of Evolutionary Psychology 5 (2007):1–4, 89–104, doi: 10.1556/JEP.2007.1010.

2   M. Schorsch, R. Gomez, T. Hahn, J. Hoelscher-Obermaier, R. Seufert, and C. Skala, "Success Rate of Inseminations Dependent on Maternal Age? An Analysis of 4246 Insemination Cycles," Geburtshilfe Frauenheilkd 73 (2013): 808–811.

3   K. Vanfraussen, I. Ponjaert-Kristoffersen, A. Brewaeys, "An Attempt to
     Reconstruct Children's Donor Concept: A Comparison between Children's and
     Lesbian Parents' Attitudes Towards Donor Anonymity," *Hum Reprod* 16 (2001):
     2019–2025.

4   P.P. Mahlstedt, K. LaBounty, W.T. Kennedy, " The Views of Adult Offspring of
     Sperm Donation: Essential Feedback for the Development of Ethical
     Guidelines within the Practice of Assisted Reproductive Technology in the
     United States," Fertil Steril 93 (2010): 2236–2246.

5   M.S. Paul, R. Berger. "Topic Avoidance and Family Functioning in Families
     Conceived with Donor Insemination," Hum Reprod 22 (2007): 2566–2571.

6   J. Howenstine, "How Systemic Enzymes Work to Cure Diseases," March 17,
     2009, http://www.newswithviews.com/Howenstine/james175.htm.

7   Hethir Rodriguez, "Study: Systemic Enzyme Therapy Promising for Recurrent
     Miscarriage," Natural Fertility Info, http://natural-fertility-info.com/enzyme-
     therapy-recurrent-miscarriage.html (Offprint from FW Dittmar, Forum
     Immunologie 3/2000).

8   J. Bledsoe and B. Johnston, "Preparing Families for International Adoption,"
     Pediatrics in Review 25 (2004).

9   T.B. Mesen, J.E. Mersereau, J.B. Kane, and A.Z. Steiner, "Optimal Timing for
     Elective Egg Freezing," Fertil Steril 103 (2015):1551–6.e1–4, doi: 10.1016/j.
     fertnstert.2015.03.002, Epub 14 Apr 2015.

10 C.C. Chang, T.A. Elliott, G. Wright, D.B. Shapiro, A.A. Toledo, and Z.P. Nagy.
     "Prospective Controlled Study to Evaluate Laboratory and Clinical Outcomes of
     Oocyte Vitrification Obtained in In Vitro Fertilization Patients Aged 30 To 39
     Years," Fertil Steril 99 (2013): 1891–1897.

11 NEW DEVELOPMENTS AND FINAL THOUGHTS

1   D.R. Meldrum, R.F. Casper, A. Diez-Juan, C. Simon, Carlos, A.D. Domar, and
     R. Frydman. "Aging and the Environment Affect Gamete and Embryo
     Potential: Can We Intervene?" *Fertil Steril* 105 (2016): 548–559.

2   K. Zaleski, "Female Company President: 'I'm sorry to all the mothers I
     worked with'," Fortune, March 3, 2015, http://fortune.com/2015/03/03/
     female-company-president-im-sorry-to-all-the-mothers-i-used-to-work-with/.

3   A. Lashinsky, "Larry Page: Google Should Be Like a Family," Fortune, January 19,
     2012, http://fortune.com/2012/01/19/larry-page-google-should-be-like-a-family/.

4   T. Rostgaard, "Family Policies in Scandinavia," Friedrich Ebert Stiftung,
     December 2014, http://library.fes.de/pdf-files/id/11106.pdf.

5   Lao Tzu, Tao Te Ching, Chapter 64.

6   R. Lewis, personal communication at a fertile soul retreat, 2004, in Austin,
     Texas. See http://www.thefertilesoul.com/.

Index

polycystic ovarian syndrome (PCOS)
(*continued*)
109, 110–11; miscarriage from, 73;
Samantha's story, 109–10, 111, 112–
14, 116, 120–21, 124; symptoms, 111
polyps, 148
polyps, endometrial, 73
poor ovarian reserve (POR), 32, 33–34,
48, 165
positive self-talk, 140–41, 141–42
positivity, 138–39
pot, 89, 95
potassium, 119
PQQ (Pyrroloquinoline quinone), 71
pre-conception treatment, 57–58, 120,
192–93, 195, 202–3. *See also* food
pregnancy: chemical, 9; monitoring at
fertility clinic, 80–81; negative self-
talk, 81; symptoms, 79–80; vaginal
bleeding, 81–83. *See also* conception
pre-implantation genetic screening
(PGS), 128, 145, 176–77
prescription medication, 98–99, 107.
See also antidepressants; drugs
pre-washed sperm, 9, 190
PRIDE program (Parent Resources for
Information, Development, and
Education), 198
progesterone, 79, 109, 156
progesterone suppositories, 81–82
prostate problems, 104, 108
protein, 13, 82, 119. *See also* meat
Public Health Agency of Canada, 51
Puragon, 126

radial artery pulse, 44
radiation, 89
red dates (Hong Zao), 15
reproductive health, *see* fertility;
fertility challenges

reproductive organs, blood flow to,
122, 123–24, 155, 195
research, personal, 77
rest, *see* sleep
retrograde ejaculation, 89, 104
rheumatoid arthritis, 138
Robertsonian translocation, *see*
chromosomal translocation
Roosevelt, Eleanor, 1
Rowling, J.K., 22
Royal Jelly, 58, 71, 191
Rubin, Lee Hullender, 61–62

salt, 119
same-sex couples, 182, 183. *See also*
female-only pregnancy; lesbian
couple
Satir, Virginia, 105
SCH (subchorionic hemorrhaging), 82
scrotum, 88, 90, 97–98
secondary infertility, 66
selenium, 101
self-care, 42–43
self-talk: negative, 81; positive, 140–41,
141–42
self-trust, 188–89
septate uterus, 73
serotonin, 55, 136
sex, *see* intercourse
sexually transmitted infections (STI),
149, 163
Shan Yao (Chinese wild yam), 15
shifts, flexible, 125, 126
shift work, 83, 118
single women, 182, 183, 192–95, 196–97,
200. *See also* female-only
pregnancy
Sjogren's disease, 129
sleep, 77, 79, 117–18
smoking, 90, 96, 107

women: desire for children, 182; energy
    life stages, 35–36; onus for fertility
    treatment on, 92–93, 99; socio-
    economic trends for, 37–38
work, 157
workplace policies: family gap in, 37;
    Google, 206–7; supportive, 121,
    122, 124–26, 206–7; unsupportive,
    112, 115, 144, 145; for young
    couples, 209

xenoestrogens, 74

yeast infections, 61

Zaleski, Katherine, 206
zinc sulfate, 101
Zuckerberg, Mark, 73